Crafting a Path Through Illness

Exploring creativity while chronically ill

Life goes by, and sets paths,
which are not travelled in vain.
… illness …
… naturally, quite often, despair …
I am still eager to live. I've started to paint again …
In spite of my long illness, I feel immense joy in
LIVING.

Frida Kahlo

Crafting a Path Through Illness

Exploring creativity while chronically ill

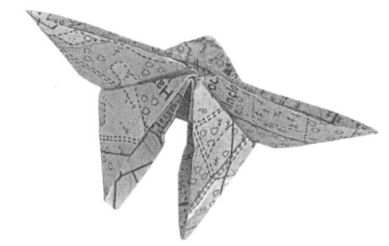

Germaine Hypher

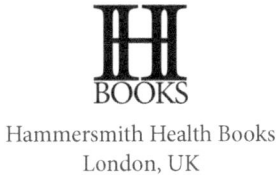

Hammersmith Health Books
London, UK

This first edition is published by Hammersmith Health Books – an imprint of Hammersmith Books Limited
4/4A Bloomsbury Square, London WC1A 2RP, UK
www.hammersmithbooks.co.uk

© 2025, Germaine Hypher (text and illustrations)

The right of Germaine Hypher has been asserted by her in accordance with the Copyright, Designs and Patents Act 1988.

All rights reserved. No part of this publication may be reproduced, stored in any retrieval system or transmitted in any form or by any means, electronic, mechanical, photocopying, recording or otherwise, without the prior permission of the publishers and copyright holder.

The information contained in this book is for educational purposes only. It is the result of the study and the experience of the author. Whilst the information and advice offered are believed to be true and accurate at the time of going to press, neither the author nor the publisher can accept any legal responsibility or liability for any errors or omissions that may have been made or for any adverse effects which may occur as a result of following the recommendations given herein. Always consult a qualified medical practitioner if you have any concerns regarding your health.

British Library Cataloguing in Publication Data: A CIP record of this book is available from the British Library.

Print ISBN 978-1-78161-266-8
Ebook ISBN 978-1-78161-267-5

Commissioning editor: Georgina Bentliff
Designed and typeset by: Julie Bennett of Bespoke Publishing Limited
Cover design by: Madeline Meckiffe
Cover image: Origami butterfly by Germain Hypher using OS Explorer OL22 New Forest Map; background by Shutterstock texture © Donatas1205
Index: Dr Laurence Errington
Production: Angela Young
Printed and bound by: TJ Books, Cornwall, UK

Contents

About the Author ix
Introduction 1
    From my path… 1
    …To yours 4

Part 1: Being ill, the creative way 7
1. A creative life 9
    Suggested creative exercise: A body of creativity 13
2. The feedback loop 15
    Suggested therapeutic activity: Art to the aid 22
3. Artistic responses to illness 23
    Suggested creative exercise: Learning from another's path 34

Part 2: Creative healthcare 35
4. An historical viewpoint 37
    Suggested therapeutic activity: A medical incantation 42
5. Crafty prescriptions for physical conditions 45
    Suggested therapeutic activity: Express yourself 51
6. Creative calm for happier health 53
    Suggested therapeutic activity: Colour wash 65

Part 3: The art of feeling larger than your illness 67
7. Creating purpose 69
    Suggested therapeutic activity: A life well lived 77
8. Making a difference 79

Suggested creative exercise: The power of you	88
9. Creative connections	91
Suggested therapeutic activity: Connections	104

Part 4: Crafting your path — 107

10. Spinning gold from straw	109
Suggested therapeutic activity: Origami butterflies	116
11. Making room for creativity	119
Suggested therapeutic activity: A creative opening ceremony	124
12. Getting the tension right	127
Suggested creative exercise: Pressure points	133
13. Stopping up the energy leaks	135
Suggested therapeutic activity: Body scan	141
14. From pushing to pacing	143
Suggested therapeutic activity: A reward jar	158
15. Good practice	161
Suggested creative exercise: A commitment certificate	170
16. Recovering from perfectionism	171
Suggested creative exercise: Embracing imperfection	179
17. Create-ability	181
Suggested creative exercise: Tools of the trade	208
18. Fallow times and beyond	211
Suggested therapeutic activity: Creative comforts	227

Part 5: A dose of inspiration — 229

19. Changing perception, not circumstance	231
Suggested creative exercises:	235
Welcoming creativity	235
How many ways?	235
Suggested therapeutic activity: Affirming your creativity	236
20. Moving with the rhythms of restriction	239
Suggested creative exercise: Repeating patterns	245
Suggested therapeutic activities	245
(Internal) weather	245
Restriction wall	246
21. Going without	249
Suggested creative exercises:	253
Attention to negative space	253

Contents

Self-denial	254
Suggested therapeutic activity: Would if I could	254
22. Going within	257
Suggested creative exercise: Follow the scent	260
Suggested therapeutic activities:	261
Self-portrait	261
Inner amulet	262
23. Listening to the voice of illness	265
Suggested creative exercises:	268
A conversation with pain (or discomfort)	268
The voice of my illness is…	269
Suggested therapeutic activity: From debris to declaration	269
24. Maximising your environment	271
Suggested creative exercises:	274
Micro-vision	274
Altering your environment	274
Suggested therapeutic activity: Creating an altar	275
25. Flights of fancy	277
Suggested creative exercises:	281
Dream journal	281
Finding a fanciful companion	282
Suggested therapeutic activity: Postcards from another reality	282
26. Borrowing from others	285
Suggested creative exercises:	287
Borrow some style	287
Take something, anything	288
Suggested therapeutic activity: Borrowing from the old and often told	288
27. Contradictions and combinations	291
Suggested creative exercises:	295
Random connections	295
Yin and yang	296
Suggested therapeutic activity: Combining contradictory views	296
28. Gathering the yarns of your life	299
Suggested creative exercises:	303
Exploring the hidden narrative	303
A guided visualisation for retrieving stories	303
Suggested therapeutic activity: Alternative translations	305

Appendices: Creative directions 307
Appendix 1. Home-friendly arts and crafts 309
Appendix 2. Charity and kindness projects 315
Appendix 3. Online resources 321
Appendix 4. Metaphors and imagery to explore 325

Bibliography 331
Acknowledgments 337
Index 339

About the Author

Germaine Hypher has been disabled by chronic illness and fatigue since childhood. She has found arts, crafts and creativity to be her constant allies, teaching her to live a well-adapted, meaningful and joyful life while predominantly unable to leave her home and often bed-based. Her writing experience has included providing content for the eco-store Natural Collection, founding and editing a nature-crafts magazine for seven years, contributions to various anthologies, winning the Hastings National Poetry Competition (2005) and winning a bursary from the Literary Consultancy. When pretending not to be as ill as she is Germaine likes to sniff the great outdoors, laugh with abandon and immerse herself in music. When illness sits on her more heavily she makes abundant use of pillows and hugs (especially of the feline and heat pad kind).

Visit www.germainehypher.weebly.com, follow @craftingapaththroughillness on Facebook and Instagram, or find Germaine Hypher on Bluesky to see a selection of her creations.

Introduction

From my path...

Rose petals, thyme leaves and toothpaste. At the end of the garden path sits a child's bucket with these ingredients steeping in water. I don't remember if it was attempting to become potion or perfume, but I do recall my childhood being all about creativity. Many childhoods are. Creativity is exploratory, unpredictable and suffused with possibility. It is the essence of childhood. If I wasn't brewing stinky concoctions, I was building a cardboard washing machine for my dolls' clothes (I wasn't devoted to my dolls but making things for them, now that was absorbing), painting plaster of Paris items, modelling with *Fimo*, French knitting, sewing, drawing or making books. Ah, making books.

I have been creating books for almost as long as I can remember. Puzzle books and poetry books, story books, illustrated factoid books about the natural world, all before I hit double figures. The only one of my handwritten creations that I still have from that time is a picture storybook inspired by the Amazonian rainforest and the cartoon, Mr Benn. It was made the same year that my body began devising its own plot twist.

At eight years old the nausea and aching joints were the first signs something was not entirely right. By 12, now experiencing a multitude of other symptoms, having stayed at Great Ormond Street Hospital for Children twice, and no longer able to attend school, a paediatrician with an electroencephalogram diagnosed childhood-onset myalgic encephalomyelitis (also known as ME/CFS – the latter letters standing for chronic fatigue syndrome, the overly simplistic and initially American moniker for the condition).

Since then, I have spent three and a half decades failing to outgrow either illness or creative play. I have learnt to navigate severe chronic illness using creativity to steer the way. This wasn't a pre-considered strategy. I was as amazed as anybody when, at 18, having assumed I just fiddled around with crafty equipment, I was awarded a place at art college. I attended a total of one day, thanks to my health.

It has frequently felt as if my body were intentionally thwarting every creative advance I attempted. I remember realising, in my late teens, just as I was discovering how much I loved nature photography, that I would not be able to indulge in it often because my muscle strength wasn't enough to hold one eye shut while I looked through the viewfinder with the other. Nor could I hold the weight of the camera without shaking the shot into a blur.

I remember lying still with my eyes shut for over 21 hours a day. I remember being spoon-fed and held up on the toilet as an adult and hearing that I risked losing my daughter to foster care because my then-husband was leaving us, while I was mostly bedbound. But my attraction to all things arty-crafty never waned, and nothing stays static. Social services, thanks to the creative thinking of a marvellous social worker, provided care so my daughter and I could stay together. My health (still very poor and fragile) began to allow me to feel, if never well, at least not as if I were expiring. Arts and crafts continually helped me to chart the terrain, smooth the path, record my experiences, and depict what I would like to have encountered more of. And digital cameras came on the scene, making photography accessible to me. Everything changes.

For years, alongside attempting to appear more well than I really was, I tried to conceal how my creative solutions were usually cobbled together from

Introduction

second-hand donations, energy-saving shortcuts and foraged household items. Instead of buying metres of desirable fabric or fancy writing books, my poetry and prose are generally composed on the backs of discarded sheets of paper, my patchwork constructed from second-hand clothing. Beads and buttons and wire and thread are rescued from disuse. Along with my body's various difficulties and my array of coping mechanisms, I now own these methods more confidently. My ideas emerge from a desire to re-use and regenerate, and a refusal to accept that something is useless or beyond redemption. I make the most of the unwanted and unrecognised, envisioning a new form of life for what is tired, rejected and resigned to redundancy. Now I come to analyse it, this reflects the way I aim to live with severe chronic illness and something I have learnt to be proud of.

So, yes, I have always played with words, yarn and scraps of fabric but, more than that, creativity, for me, is a way of life. Creative fixes, mends and alternatives help me live ecologically, frugally and as fully as possible within my confined arena. Creativity brings me enjoyment and provides me with a sense of purpose. It acknowledges and calms my demons. It connects me with others. I think it has become my *raison d'être*.

> *We all have at least one personal creative superpower, even if it takes a lifetime to discover it.*

Still mostly housebound, and frequently in close communion with a bed, it becomes apparent that not only is a creative approach to life my personal super-power (we all have at least one, even if it takes a lifetime to discover) but that there are many others out there like me. Some are feeling as isolated and uniquely disabled by illness as I so often have.

I'm here to tell you that I have suggestions for making the experience more creatively negotiable. If you feel that, in some small measure, my words could help, then please read on. We'll craft this path together.

...to yours

If you, too, live with a disabling chronic condition, sometimes you will face a brick wall of illness. Despite your every effort, it simply will not allow you to advance in your chosen direction. Career, social life, hobbies will feel stolen away. This is not the end of your story. It is an opportunity for a sub-plot or twist to come forth.

Just for now, accept that the wall exists. Stop repeatedly walking into it like a clueless zombie, exhausting yourself with fruitless efforts. Equally, try not to be intimidated by the solidity of it looming over you and blocking the view. Instead, slow down. Look along this boundary for any murals or graffitied stories to entertain or guide you. There may be a decorated tunnel underneath the wall or a seat alongside it on which you can take time to recoup some energy and learn new skills while you wait awhile. Is that an art box and sewing basket left there for just such a person as you? Do you perhaps spy another path leading away from or around the wall? Think creatively. Consider a deliberate, rather than enforced, change of focus. Whether you one day knock down that wall or remain this side of it, decorating it in your own style, only the future knows.

Sometimes both contentment and deeper creativity come from accepting our limitations and examining them for what they offer, rather than what they deprive us of. This is not to be confused with giving up. Accepting the gravity of your physical situation, working compassionately with it, and embracing the many aspects of yourself is the best thing you can do for yourself.

When symptoms are given space to exist without concealment or denial, we paradoxically feel more in control. We can learn to own our experiences through expressing ourselves in whatever creative form we most connect with. We may even develop the confidence to connect with others by sharing our experience artistically.

Introduction

Perhaps glimpses of creativity compel you but you cannot quite find the right route. Maybe you are already treading an artistic path but struggling to traverse it with new symptoms. Or have you never previously considered yourself creative but find yourself wondering if new circumstances call for new practices?

What can you do to awaken inspiration and nurture creativity?

First, think carefully about where you want to be looking. Focus on what you *do* have, not what you don't. Recognise opportunities and raw materials in your life that you might previously have paid scant attention to. Where can you set your sights now? What creative hobby might you enjoy that you have not tried before or haven't picked up in a long while? What can you make from the remnants of life as you knew it?

> *Focus on what you* **do** *have rather than what you don't.*

Sometimes, with a little lateral thinking, some simple engineering of what is in front of you, and a dose of imagination, there *is* a way. This is the path I want to explore with you.

It is demoralising when our body rebels against whatever we ask of it. When such feelings threaten to overwhelm you, take heart that, however slow and subtle, change is always on the horizon. Options come into view; fresh interests supersede initial choices; what you cannot manage now you may well achieve later. I am still discovering tools and techniques that allow me to practise previously inaccessible hobbies.

At times, we all need ideas, assistance and a reminder that our creative pursuits are enough. We need a sense of community and role models to make us aware of how dreams can become possibilities. With limited physical resources we are keen to know that how we choose to spend our time may also benefit our health. Whether you are nurturing an artistic leaning, looking for new hobbies after being felled by illness, or wanting to express the effects of chronic illness more creatively, through this book I hope to help you.

I can't offer kits for banishing symptoms or make every craft accessible to you. The term disabled would be irrelevant if there were always a simple solution, and some chronic illness symptoms can be disabling to the absolute extreme – incapacitating not just a portion of the body but the whole system. I am also acutely aware of the offence that generalised advice can cause, so please bear in mind that whatever I say is only what I have found to be of benefit to myself or those I've connected with. Dip in and out of these pages as they appeal to you. There is no great need to read them en masse in chronological order. I'm relying on you to take what serves you and leave the rest for someone else (perhaps a future you).

If not already, you will become the expert on your own body's manifestation of your condition and how you can expand your life creatively. Time, trial and error will teach you where your forté lies and the boundaries to work within. You will learn from others as well as from your unique presentations of your illness. Listen to this expertise you hold and act wisely. While being attentive to the rules of your experience, allow yourself to imagine beyond the usual. If it's within your safe capabilities, do what feels good and make what pleases you, regardless of what others may think or say. Being comfortably content with yourself and your own creative life is what matters on this adventure.

So, ask yourself what *you* want to work with, what *you* want to create, and *how* you can achieve this. Make mistakes and take a break (that bit's important); try again, think new thoughts and adapt to suit your needs. This is where creativity begins.

Part 1:
Being ill, the creative way

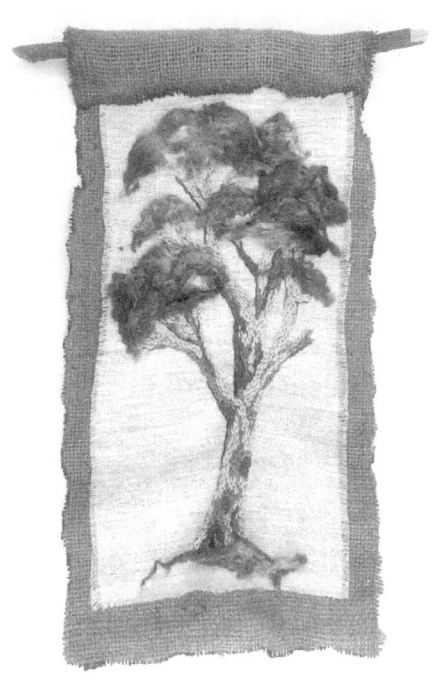

Chapter 1
A creative life

When chronically ill, we must find gentle and rewarding ways to occupy ourselves. Arts and crafts are just such occupations that we can turn to. We may startlingly realise that creativity was within us all along, side-lined by a previously hectic life, but what if creativity doesn't feel natural to you?

Let me reassure you.

Creativity is intrinsic to being human. We all absorb what is around us and use what we experience as the building blocks for self-expression and our chosen path through life. Some people do this more reflexively than thoughtfully, some with more original perceptions but, ultimately, we are all creators. If you are doubting whether you have what it takes to play imaginatively with arts and crafts, consider this: we all make something from the days that we wake into, we all manifest dreams when we sleep (whether we remember them or not), we are all the artists of our own lives.

Life itself is a creative process. And yet I have often heard people bemoan their lack of creativity. They may knit, cook interesting meals, garden, think of ways to spread kindness, enjoy photography, find new methods of fundraising for charities, but assume they're not creative because they don't produce original works of art. If you are enjoying coming up with something from the ingredients of your life, that is creative. For this moment, dive in fully so that whatever you produce is a little piece of you.

> *If you are enjoying coming up with something from the ingredients of your life, that is creative.*

Feeling like we don't belong or aren't enough is common when living in the hidden sickroom-edges of society, but there is a place for everything and everyone; for you and whatever you bring into being. Engaging in whatever creative process is within reach is a powerful affirmation of your unique ability to create an experience of your own making. We can make peace with our place in the world by filling our own corner of existence with any manner of creativity, whether it is saleable or personally therapeutic, original or derivative, created for sheer joy or because a problem necessitated it.

Creativity's relationship with health

Those who have spent time with chronic illness are prone to uncovering their creative side, partly for the simple reason that sedentary hobbies are generally accessible. When removed in so many ways from the usual aspects of life, the desire to feel like we are actively living, as opposed to just existing, becomes an insistent urge. Creativity goes some way to fulfilling this need. We want to occupy our fidgety fingers and curious minds when stuck at home, or in hospital wards and waiting rooms, and handcrafts fit the bill. But there are other instigators of this relationship, too.

Inventive solutions to day-to-day problems must be found when society hasn't paved the way for our individual needs. By default, we learn that creative thinking works for us.

Meanwhile, difficult states associated with long-term health issues – isolation, loss of identity, longing, grief, injustice and physical pain – all find a therapeutic outlet in the arts.

We may be looking to re-create something lost to us or to make more visible that which is paid scarce attention or poorly understood. We don't want to live with a haunting absence or the feeling of not being recognised, so the void created when our health declines must be addressed. We can fill it with less than healthy habits or we can mine it for creative presence. Like Victorian botanists, we travel through the foreign lands of our struggles to bring back curiosities and new sensations.

Creativity is a healthy coping mechanism when dealing with limitation and pain. Innovative musings pass the time, distract from less healthy ruminations, train the brain to see the world more constructively and transform the mundane. Even if images and ideas never move into the physical world, they are still valuable. I have come up with countless ideas that will only ever exist in my mind. They might have been disastrous had I attempted them. We need never know. I have entertained myself with their imagined existence and strengthened my creative thinking skills every time I've indulged in creative fantasy. Creativity – be it your own or an admired artist's – invites a rich inner world to recline in.

Creativity as an ally

Creativity is a fun ally. It helps us pay attention to the curved path that travels sometimes around and other times deeply into limitations. It encourages us to embrace questions as much as answers. *What can I do with this? What would happen if…? How can I…?* It nurtures unusual responses and frequently holds hands with both the sublime and the ridiculous but never feels an obligation to be either. It is eternally curious.

We can see our inner creator at work when we want to communicate but extreme fatigue or cognitive impairment prevents us from remembering even basic words and our brain automatically circumnavigates the lost word to find a new way of expressing itself. 'The potatoes need folding,' I have said because it at least started with the same letter as pillowcases and had a similar sound pattern to it. Where I used to try to hide my cognitive difficulties or would become fixated on remembering the correct word, distressing myself the further I failed, I now celebrate the creative alternatives my brain comes up with. I have learned that if I open

Creativity, hidden within and driven by the plot of our life, helps us step towards transformation.

the door to a different outcome then something interesting will often reveal itself.

When learning creative writing skills, we are taught that the basis of plot is conflict followed by resolution, with the protagonist being changed en route. Creativity, hidden within and driven by the plot of our life, helps us make that step towards transformation. What in your life's current plotline is calling for transformation? A house into a home, a garden into a sanctuary, scraps into a blanket, a blank page into self-expression, or a health limitation into a fulfilling life? Perhaps you feel driven to make items to fill a space in someone's world, raise awareness, or inspire a different perspective? These are all examples of a creative life well lived.

Imagining creativity into existence

The artist Riva Lehrer, who was born with spina bifida and spent a lifetime navigating the difficulties that came with her condition, asserts that imagination is at the very core of living with disability. And before you tell me that you're not particularly imaginative, let me ask if you've ever feared the worst, living viscerally with the many potentials of a scenario that never came to pass. That's imagination at work. It takes practice to harness this constructively, but the raw materials are already there inside you.

Creativity needn't be a unique concept or rare talent. Open yourself up to the possibility that you might have more capacity for creativity than you previously considered. What feels obvious or easy to you may not be apparent to someone else so don't scrimp on expressing yourself creatively just because you take for granted what comes naturally to you. 'It *doesn't* come naturally to me, that's my problem,' you might be thinking. So hear this – creativity can be bought, taught and developed. Allow your natural imagination to play with this realisation and have a go.

Have a go at responding to other people's creativity. Using craft kits, colouring books, or music composed by others doesn't negate your own creative input. Kits guide the hands while the brain establishes skill and mulls over ideas. Choosing which shades to use on an intricate colouring-in page exercises your aesthetic autonomy. Whether you are re-telling old stories, playing other musician's compositions or stitching a commercial pattern you are breathing new life – your own life – into a creative tradition.

Pre-packaged creative activities take you from imagining the existence of an item to the actualisation of it: a real thing to have and to hold – made by you! They are a way to put yourself into a creation without feeling too emotionally exposed or daunted by the whole concept of where to start. They are a gentle form of making when symptoms are too strong to allow you to focus on originality and they lend themselves to adaptation as your skills and confidence develop. If there's one thing those disabled by chronic conditions are good at it is adaptation, and that is when you realise you are more imaginative than you gave yourself credit for.

Admittedly, at times my imagination has shown itself to be worse than shy. My visualisation skills are poor and my fatigued brain often lacks the energy to stretch itself far, collapsing instead into nearby clichés, but I have learnt to look beyond the familiar and to gently lean into my creative thinking skills. In later chapters I'll be sharing practical advice on how you too can do this.

When we practise using our imagination it becomes a more natural habit. We learn not to turn automatically to the obvious but to embrace the unexpected in both life and art. This doesn't always work out as we imagined but it is all part of the creative path.

Suggested creative exercise
A body of creativity

Recall the ways you have been creative throughout your life. If it feels affirming for you, write them down or create a collage that represents your creative life so far. Include childhood games and projects, styling your appearance, cooking, decorating your home, telling inventive fibs, daydreaming, problem solving, and anything else remotely creative.

To better acquaint yourself with your creative self, complete the following sentences:

> I feel most creative when…
> I feel least creative when…
> I can help myself to be more creative by…
> I feel inspired by…

A creative life at a glance

- Creativity is not something that only gifted artists and crafters possess. It is at the core of our being.
- It is a natural human response to turn to creativity to problem-solve, draw strength, pass time and bring comfort.
- Illness and disability predispose us to thinking up creative solutions to our difficulties.
- We can exercise our creative muscle to develop its strength.

Chapter 2
The feedback loop

Your creative self does not live in a vacuum. It is part and parcel of who you are, lending itself to and drawing upon various aspects of your being. Cross-referencing your creative developments and achievements with the way you manage your health and choose to experience your chronic illness can bring greater rewards to both.

Life is a work of art

Just as it takes perseverance to become proficient in any craft, it takes time and effort to adjust to a body's unique pains and limitations. Like the mysterious abbreviations of a knitting pattern, chronic illness requires you to learn signs and methods and to work with what you've been given. You are becoming an adept. If you could perceive living with chronic illness as just another craft, one that frequently comes without a well-written set of instructions, would you feel prouder of what you are making of your life? The Middle English definition of art was 'a skill that comes about as a result of learning or practice'. By this definition, our very lives are works in progress. So let's, as Nietzsche said, 'Make life a work of art'.

We can shape our chosen identity just as we mould and sketch and stitch our craft. When we mix colours and combine words, we practise the art of creating satisfaction from disparate elements, reminding ourselves of the importance of even the smallest inclusion. While we take apart old garments to re-use in textile art or fashion design, we prime ourselves to unpick old, redundant life ideas, reshaping them to fit our current circumstances. As we use materials for novel purposes, or tweak existing patterns, we learn the value of re-styling our partially functioning bodies into new forms of efficacy. Over time, we embellish our days with tiny, exquisite joys. By working creatively towards a result within our reach, our brain develops greater faith in future adaptive successes.

Responding artistically to our situation, perhaps acquiring greater objectivity along the way, we are better enabled to either accommodate our illness or to recognise that which we have the power to adjust. We practise, we learn, we adapt our techniques or plans. Our thread tangles, snaps or refuses to go where we want it. We glue our fingers together. Colours that we chose don't combine well. Clichés abound in our writing, plots refuse to develop, failures accrue.

So we try again.

We reach around until we find the form of expression that best suits us. And we create something. Perhaps something small or amateur, but it is an achievement.

Similarly, our body may not reach where we'd intended. It may wobble, not look 'normal' or do the things we think it should. But we now have the insight and creativity to develop constructive coping mechanisms and calm strategies to aid either recovery or acceptance of a more permanent condition. Along with creative offerings, we are crafting ourselves and in turn we are feeding our reservoir of creative integrity.

The good...

When you feel happy with your work, snuggle up to that feeling during your post-exertion recuperation and let it stroke you into happy restfulness. Later, when you are ready to think more actively, ask yourself what you are most proud of in that piece or your execution of it. What is it that makes it succeed in what you set out to do? Celebrate your ability to manifest this and lodge it in your brain so you can draw on that skill again in the future. Be specific about what you have achieved and how you can transfer these skills into other areas of your life.

Did you slow down and work with extra care this time, discovering that you made fewer mistakes and worked more effectively when you paced and rested, despite the desire to push onwards without pause? Did taking that break for an hour, a day, a week or months not destroy the flow of your work, as you had feared, but enhance the end product by allowing you to slowly accumulate more ideas and absorb fresh stimuli? Maybe you could similarly benefit from not urgently rushing to attend to your mind's whirring thoughts or other people's demands on your energy.

Did you learn to trust that the outcome would make the time spent on it worthwhile? In the future, when other activities seem so much more alluring than bedrest or physiotherapy, will this experience remind you of the value of dedication to the future goal?

Did you accept that the outcome need not be how you imagined it and that the unexpected can be better than the idea you originally dreamt up? Perhaps this will make it easier for you to cope with the disappointments that chronic illness can generate.

Have you discovered adaptive dexterity techniques that can be applied to other activities? Do you now have more confidence in your ability to learn something new and accomplish what you find hard or laborious? Perhaps taking on board a different perspective or amalgamating different techniques resulted in a satisfying finished piece. Could a similarly broadened outlook in other areas of life better help you to discover solutions to some difficulties or symptoms?

Accept that the outcome need not be how you imagined it and that the unexpected can be better than the idea you originally dreamt up.

Perhaps your artistic expression solidified amorphous feelings, releasing concepts that could assist your communication skills with healthcare professionals, friends and family?

Finding ourselves capable in a field of creativity that had initially felt daunting is a wonderful reminder of possibilities. Are you similarly able to do more within the confines of your chronic illness than was at first apparent? This needn't mean travelling further along your pre-illness path. It means heeding your health's insistence and looking at other, more imaginative and subtle, ways to make the most of life. It means finding the creative joys that your previous trajectory hadn't highlighted.

…The bad…

Just as you can integrate your creative successes into the way you live your wider life, your messes and muddles can also be instructive, teaching you how to handle frustration and recognise alternative options. Chronic illness so often feels all-encompassing, sucking our life into its hungry orbit until we feel out of control and at a loss as to how to be content with what remains. The stakes are so high that it is hard to think objectively and balance our responsive emotions. One failed creative idea or pared down project doesn't carry this weight with it. It is easier to develop constructively adaptive strategies, modified approaches, and emotionally healthy reactions to perceived failures in the world of craft than it is to accept broader disappointments. Once you have begun to do this, it may become more obvious how to integrate these patterns of thought into the way you deal with bigger problems in life. A happy by-product of processing reactions to life events via creativity is that it will serve both your emotional self and the creations that result from this synthesis.

Of course, sometimes it will be your creativity that doesn't turn out how you'd like and here the feedback loop can come full circle, with your health providing helpful examples. A life with chronic illness undoubtedly feels far from perfect, and you may have crumpled at some point, but you haven't given up. The fact that you're reading or listening to this demonstrates that you have begun to unfurl at the edges and feel the hand of fortitude smoothing you out. You are here, making the most of the creative life force that sits sculpting motivation just beneath your visible surface. Recognition of your resilience, as well as other constructive traits, can inform your approach to your involvement in the world of arts and crafts.

…And the undervalued

We tend to take for granted not just what comes naturally to us but that which we've practised until it feels innate. When I'm responding to somebody's praise of a teddy or blanket I've knitted, I have to stop myself from muttering, 'but it's nothing. I just followed the pattern/combined different stitches'. I remind myself how I used to look at other people's similar creations in awe. I make myself recall the first few times I saw a knitting pattern and my brain tumbled over itself trying to understand this new language and what all the abbreviations could possibly mean. Over time it became easier until I almost forgot the learning process I'd been through, but to dismiss this is to do ourselves a disservice.

Similarly, when people observe that the way you cope with your illness is 'so brave' or 'inspiring", try not to leap to denial. Yes, bravery is a choice, and you might have little choice but to live with your condition, but you do get to choose *how* you live with it. That is what the praise is for.

> *You have little choice but to live with your condition but you do get to choose* **how** *you live with it.*

Our abilities and levels of tolerance loop and curve. We develop, forget, remember and refine them over time. When they combine to create something pleasing, receive the praise graciously. You've earned it.

But what about when praise isn't forthcoming? How do we cope when society or loved ones don't recognise the effort we are putting into crafting a successful life with a disabling illness, or when our foray into handmade treasures isn't valued? We must give ourselves credit for getting where we are and achieving the skills we have acquired. Along the way we may have embarked on crafts that we simply could not get the hang of (don't ever ask me to sculpt a likeness in clay) and may have tried health strategies, cures and responses that didn't serve us in the long run. But what about the strategies and attempts that did pay off, if only in small ways and the passing of days?

Let us take stock of our mini-triumphs and be proud to exhibit them – to proclaim our strengths and fresh achievements – and help others to recognise our daily efforts, creative or otherwise. It probably feels like life itself forced these developments, delivering more and more tangles and life-splodges to be dealt with. But it was we who kept rummaging around until we found what we could best work with and how to use it. We didn't give up on the larger craft of living creatively. Every small act built upon another, feeding back into both our craft-life and general existence.

It can help to remember that the value of a creation or situation is not dependent on the outcome. The Dalai Lama teaches that Tibetans value a piece of art, not by its appearance but how the creator experienced the making of it and the internal changes they underwent.

If you are finding it hard to find any merit in your creative offerings or, indeed, in yourself, and you have a sneaking suspicion that you chronically undervalue what you offer to the world, you may find it constructive to turn to Chapter 16: Recovering from perfectionism, in Part 4.

Looking up close at the collage of life

What you conjure from the opportunities and materials available to you is all part of the mixed media collage of your life. Whether you share your creations or keep them for your eyes only, they pay homage to life itself, bearing witness to individual and collective experiences. It is wise, therefore, to pay close attention to the different aspects of life and how they can best be honoured.

We learn, when our days become focused under the magnifying glass of chronic illness, that there is less room for unnecessary life-clutter or fussing over external achievements. Instead, we find a greater need for clarity about what we really want our days to contain. We are better equipped when we look through that lens with curiosity rather than kneejerk judgement. Yes, we will see the irregularities of ill health and the shadows of erased abilities, but we will also be rewarded by intricate detail and easily missed observations.

Each day we can practise adjusting our expectations – of our bodies and of art. We can take time to consider what we might learn to find attractive, interesting, or at least acceptable, by shifting the lens to another angle and bringing new perspectives into view. Our wiggle room may not be vast, but we still have choices in how to outgrow the restrictions of a fixed viewpoint or limited appreciation.

Acknowledge the limitations you can't ignore while exploring what new associations and patterns you *can* work with, in your creations and your wider life. Bring your focus in and out, experimenting with where on the continuum of minimalism and maximalism you best exist. Look for a resting place that reflects your nature while simultaneously respecting your health needs and stretching your creative muscle. Then ask yourself how these can inform and benefit each other.

> *We are better equipped if we look through the lens of chronic illness with curiosity rather than kneejerk judgement.*

Creatively affirming our strengths and accepting our limitations, we acknowledge where we are and what we are capable of while discovering how best to express and fulfil our needs and emotions. Meanwhile, our physical difficulties can guide our creative path, opening new channels to shape our creativity. In the following chapter we will learn how others have found this to be the case.

Suggested therapeutic activity
Art to the aid

Choose an aid, or any object, that helps you live with your illness, and allow it to have a conversation with your creative side. Personalise a wheelchair with a cushion, fairy lights or wheel-guards. Decorate a walking stick, frame or crutches with paint, stickers, decals, transfers or rhinestones and a glue gun. Make an individual holder for your disability parking badge, or an attractive stoma pouch cover. Liven up whatever equipment your chronic illness necessitates so that it loses some of its resented medical associations and becomes a more pleasurable extension of you. In this way, your craftiness influences life with medical needs, while your health broadens your creative outlet.

The feedback loop at a glance

- Living well with chronic illness is an art in itself.
- We can cross-reference what we learn through our creative exploits with what we learn from our illness, using this knowledge to enhance both aspects of our life.
- Frustrations of crafting disasters are less emotionally charged than those related to our health. We can learn from them how to better handle stronger emotions and to value what we *can* do.
- Examining life as if it were a work of art helps us to discover new perceptions.
- Through decorating our disability aids we can encourage our physicality and our creativity to influence each other.

Chapter 3
Artistic responses to illness

Arts and crafts exert a widely beneficial effect on the lives of all who enjoy them, but for people with disabling health conditions they can prove particularly adaptable and therapeutic. There is also evidence throughout history of ill health proffering fresh perspectives that the world of arts has benefited from.

That, however, is not the whole picture. I do not want to romanticise ill health or suggest that everyone can partake in artistic or creative activities, nor that all have the inclination to do so. Some artists have been known to have long periods of inactivity due to their health. The poet **Rainer Maria Rilke** spent a number of years ill with leukaemia, before it took his life, unable to write any poetry at all. Drafts of two of his famous poems were left abandoned during this time. **Dostoyevsky's** epilepsy influenced his writing but immediately after a seizure he would feel drained and listless, unable to write or even read for a few days 'because I am a wreck, body and soul'. Similarly, **Virginia Woolf** had times in bed when she couldn't write for weeks on end. Other artists, such as **Paul Klee** and **Raoul Dufy**, found their rigid, painful joints (caused, respectively, by scleroderma and arthritis) impeded fluidity, detail and exuberance in their paintings. If you are in a health crash that has pushed creative pursuits beyond your reach, take heart that great artists have experienced the same and many have come out the other side.

> *Tenacity, adaptability, talent and motivation can rise with the flames of illness.*

For now, let's enjoy spending some time with artists whose physical constraints contributed to their artistic expression. Some found that their health removed them from their original life trajectory, providing an opportunity to explore a latent talent, others that painful experiences demanded artistic expression in order to cope emotionally. Many adapted their chosen craft to suit their needs or branched into a divergent arena. This ability to transpose creative skill from one medium or body part to another is more readily understandable when we know that memories for different learned actions are not stored in specific areas of the brain but spread throughout. This seems to allow for a greater transfer of abilities when necessary.

It is inspiring to see what tenacity, adaptability, talent and motivation can rise with the flames of illness and how art can foster a greater sense of wellbeing within the parameters of chronic ill health.

Visual artists

The Spanish painter **Francisco Goya** suffered from multiple health issues resulting in depression, weight loss and deafness. While his earlier works realistically depicted what he saw, as his health deteriorated, and he came to paint more for himself than on commission, his paintings took on more imaginative characteristics. Circumstances beyond his control had affected his internal equilibrium and sensory input, instigating a more personal style and breaking him free from convention. According to the art historian **Tobi Zausner**, where his paintings had previously been dominated by bright colours he now included dark shadows, lending more power and structure to the images.

Claude Monet, although not living with an incurable chronic illness, exemplifies the link between 'faulty' senses and fresh creativity. His later paintings of the same subject matter as his earlier ones show a dramatic change in his perception of colour and his ability to see clearly. His failing eyesight caused him (in his own words) to 'see everything in a fog', with most colours filtered out by his cataracts so that everything took on a red hue. A successful operation enabled Monet to view this change in his work, leaving him horrified at his inaccurate renditions. He regarded these later pieces as ugly and went so far as to destroy some of them. Despite this personal rejection of his body's influence on his art, others saw something new and exciting in his altered visions. What remained of Monet's later works went on to have a positive impact on the onset of abstract art, expressionism and the subsequent development of art.

Prior to Monet, **Vincent van Gogh** was also producing artwork that shared how his body was interpreting the world around him. As well as being born with a brain lesion, he is believed to have suffered from acute intermittent porphyria and temporal lobe epilepsy. It's thought that his doctor prescribed digitalis, which is now known to cause yellow spots in one's vision, to help with the related seizures. This has led art historians to speculate on how much his health and medication influenced his propensity for working with the colour yellow. It is also suggested that his distinctive depiction of the sky in *Starry Night* may have been inspired by the halos of light his swollen retinas could have caused him to see around lit objects. Van Gogh also lived with bipolar disorder, and his manic phases were instrumental in his prolific artistic output.

It is hard to imagine modern art without the vivid colours and patterns of **Henri Matisse** and yet his intended career was in the legal profession. It was only during a year's hiatus from his workplace, due to appendicitis, that he began painting as a way of occupying himself and thus discovered his artistic talent. Later in life, his health was severely affected when surgery for colon cancer left him predominantly bedbound and reliant on a wheelchair. Rather than considering this the end of his artistic abilities, he adapted his techniques to suit his new limitations and invented his now iconic cut-out series. Using chalk attached to the end of a stick to draw outlines on the wall, he directed where he wanted his paper shapes to be applied. Matisse regarded this period as his second life, embracing the opportunity to reconsider his priorities and experience beauty via his own artwork.

Born later than Matisse but dying in the same year, **Frida Kahlo** was also using art to respond to her health conditions. Although she is famously known for her severe injuries and over 32 operations, resulting from both childhood polio and a road accident, what is less well publicised is the fact that she was born with spina bifida. It was this painful condition that often confined her to bed. Like Matisse, Kahlo found a way to express her artistic self from her bed. Lying flat on her back, she had an easel designed to fit over her body. For her, who famously asserted that she painted out of necessity, this was a vital aid. Her depictions of her own physical and emotional pain are her strongest legacy. Pain is also the cause of her move from a meticulous style to looser marks when medication unsteadied her hands.

Paul Smith's name may not be as recognisable as the artists mentioned so far, but his work is no less exciting. Throughout seven decades of creating art while living with cerebral palsy, he became known as the 'Typewriter Artist'. The severity of his condition meant that he found it difficult to hold a pen, pencil, pastel crayon or paintbrush and, due to speech difficulties, was limited in ways of expressing himself. Refusing to stay trapped within himself, he searched for a way to let his artistic side out. After initially playing with an old typewriter at the age of 11, he learnt to create phenomenal pictures with just one finger and the symbol keys on the top row. Using these keys to build up marks and shading on the paper, and a selection of typewriter ribbons for a limited colour palette, he would spend weeks and even months on an individual piece of art, resulting in pictures that astonish with their artistic merit, only revealing their innovative origin when viewed close up.

Rather than trying to ignore her brain scans she could take back some control by using the medium of art to transform them into something beautiful.

Elizabeth Jameson is a contemporary artist whose illness has also been instrumental in the use of unusual resources as a basis for art. Now known as the 'MRI Alchemist', her foray into this branch of creativity began when she was in the process of being diagnosed with multiple sclerosis (MS). At first, she couldn't look at her brain scans, finding the sterility of them ugly and frightening. However, she realised that rather than trying to ignore them she could take back some control by using the medium of art to transform them into something beautiful. She went on to use her scans to inspire vividly coloured copper etchings and embroideries. Now a quadriplegic, Elizabeth still creates art, using her voice to guide an assistant who does the manual work for her.

Writers

Gustave Flaubert may be cited as a literary great, but his finished pieces belie the difficulties his health placed on his urge to write. He lived with a rare form of epilepsy that severely impinged on his ability to find the words he was seeking. The original handwritten manuscripts of his creations, containing many more crossed out and rejected words than the ones that remain in his published work, show how hard he had to work to express his creative ideas in the way he desired.

Lewis Carroll used the effects of his migraines so successfully in his writing that the condition he was living with came to be named after his most famous piece of work. His unusual type of migraine caused hallucinations that distorted his perception of his body's size and shape. No doubt it's becoming clear to you how these experiences inspired him, and as more became known about his condition it was named Alice in Wonderland syndrome.

Flannery O'Connor lived with the autoimmune disease lupus. While she undoubtedly missed out on much that others around her were able to do, her writings imply that she didn't see her condition as preventing her from experiencing life's deepest lessons or inspirations. Instead, she asserted that, despite having been nowhere other than the state of illness, being sick was a place of its own, delivering more lessons than any long geographical travels. Her illness used up almost all of her energy, forcing her to ration the moments she could spend writing but this only made her appreciate and closely observe those moments all the more. When she was feeling a little better after one particularly ill spell, she worked for an hour a day, claiming to savour those moments like a fine meal.

Laura Hillenbrand was so unwell with ME when writing her bestselling novel *Seabiscuit* that she could only formulate a paragraph or two a day. At times this had to be done from her bed and even, when the dizziness triggered by focusing her eyes became too much to bear, with her eyes shut. Despite the mammoth ways in which her body was causing her pain, discomfort and limitation, she found that when inhabiting her characters she was able to temporarily forget about the severity of her symptoms.

Susanna Clark developed CFS part way through her writing career. Her first novel, *Dr Strange and Mr Norrell*, required research, complex creative decisions and a quantity of writing that was now beyond her abilities. Rather than feeling defeated by what she could no longer do, she made the decision to simplify her expectations of herself. At times she had to write *Piranesi*, her award-winning second novel that metaphorically echoes aspects of living with an isolating condition, in bursts of no more than 20 minutes due to her limited energy levels. Even after the book's completion, she still finds herself benefiting from the creation of its protagonist whose sense of belonging in the setting she created for him reminds her that being confined to a limited existence needn't equal an unhappy life.

Claire Wade became ill with severe ME at 10 years old. 'To cope with being in a darkened room 24 hours a day I started imagining my own stories. The escapism was a lifeline and without realising it I took the first steps towards becoming an author.' Although still living with her condition, its improvement allowed her to put her imaginative explorations out into the world, resulting in winning a publishing contract for her first novel, *The Choice*. 'I love the fact that writing gives me a voice and the freedom to explore a world my body physically can't,' she says. As well as expressing her own creativity, Claire pioneers for disability awareness and equality in the world of literature in a bid to dismantle the barriers many disabled authors face.

Jessica Taylor-Bearman has published a trilogy of memoirs about her experience of very severe ME. When in hospital for four years, unable to feed herself and barely able to speak, she kept an audio diary, recording a handful of words a day. 'It was exhausting. I would literally spend the whole day thinking about what sentence I wanted to say.' This not only helped her communicate that she was still herself inside her immobile body, but also formed the basis for her first book that she wrote years later when back home, having regained some use of her body. 'I write because, while I don't expect anyone to understand, I want to feel represented,' she explains.

Another way Jessica found of expressing her creative self was something she has named 'laughter painting'. Caregivers placed a lap easel, canvas and paints on her prone body in bed and rested a paintbrush in her hand. With her arm supported, Jessica then dipped the brush into the colour of her choice. Her caregiver would say things to make her laugh while the paintbrush made contact with the canvas. Whatever movement the laughter caused the paintbrush to make on the canvas became part of the artwork. Through this technique, Jessica has produced impressive landscapes that artistically incorporate, rather than sidestepping, her situation.

Composers and musicians

Had it not been for **Antonio Vivaldi's** chronic asthma preventing him from leading mass, he would have entered the priesthood, and the world might never have gained his musical compositions. Instead, his health relegated his role in the church to that of choir master, followed by musical director, giving him the opportunity to better explore his musical talents.

Niccolo Paganini, known as Demon of Fiddlers due to his virtuoso violin playing, was born with Ehlers-Danlos syndrome (EDS). His hyper-mobile joints, caused by this condition, enabled him to play the violin in his famously remarkable way. His left wrist moved so flexibly in all directions that he could perform flourishes that could be considered the musical signature of his disorder. There is surely more to Paganini's talent than mere loose joints, and EDS brings with it other symptoms of a less helpful nature, but there's no denying that his health contributed to his unique musical flair.

Gustav Mahler, when diagnosed with a heart defect, developed acute anxiety. This became a long-term condition that troubled him greatly. However, he found he was able to channel it constructively when transforming the nervous energy into popular music and composing musical scores. Without this response to his condition, and the ramifications of chronic anxiety, would we have his symphonies today?

In their own words

Moving our attention away from the public arena is just as interesting as delving into the backgrounds of famous artists. Perhaps more so, as we can allow ourselves to identify with those who regard themselves as creative but aren't held up as icons. We can imagine ourselves in their company, sharing experiences, ideas and emotional responses.

So, imagine now, sitting in a comfy chair or curled up on a floor cushion at a creativity group for those with chronic illness. Perhaps you, along with some others, are tucked up in your own bed, joining in via an internet feed. Feel the solidarity around you, the understanding. The disparate coping strategies and inspirations slide close enough to each other to create new generations of ideas. What do some of the other members of this group have to say about their relationship with creativity and chronic illness?

Christina initiates the chat by telling us what creativity means to her. 'Creativity is my happy place. I live with a very energy-limiting illness which makes "visiting" this place inconsistent, unpredictable, and oftentimes not possible at all. When I'm able to create – whether it be art, baking, jewellery-making, or any act of bringing something into existence from my imagination – it takes me to an expansive state of mind that feels free with no limits. That's something very refreshing to feel when you don't experience it physically. Time seems to operate differently here too, as it always escapes me. That's of course until the symptoms of my body rudely interrupt. They call me back down and demand I stop and rest; a very hard thing to do when it's the last thing I want to do. In the meantime, I think of ideas for my next "visit", whenever my health allows it to happen.'

Kiri is a keen nature photographer who knows all too well about waiting for one's body to be able to engage in creative passions. She has had to find other ways to explore her desire to interact creatively with the natural world since her health deteriorated. Now, she says, 'I take inspiration from my garden and the view through the bedroom window of the seasons turning, which I take snaps of using my mobile phone.' With these as a reference, she uses watercolour pens and pencils to create a nature journal, which she shares with us today. A pastoral scene borders the top of one page. Lower down, close-up depictions of toadflax and comfrey flowers surround hand-written text. A speckled-wood butterfly has been painted using a dry-resist medium with a colour wash over the top. 'I keep my drawings mostly very small and simple. Adding text to the page reduces space to fill,' she says as she guides our eyes over the page. 'I use dry coloured pencils if too fatigued, but if I choose watercolour pencils, I can activate with water later, so it's quite flexible with pacing. I aim for one page a month but do it slowly over time, without worrying if too ill to complete it or if I need to skip it.'

Sara agrees about the need to be flexible in how she expresses herself. Referring to *Hungry Little Shadow*, a puppet film she has made and shared for people to watch for free on YouTube, she says, 'I planned to perform this piece as a solo show in small cafe spaces. When my increasing symptoms made that too much to contemplate, I thought these puppets would stay shut up in a suitcase in the attic forever. The chance to pivot to a digital presentation of this piece has allowed me to breathe life into it in a way I couldn't have imagined when I began. I was able to create this show in a way that was accessible to my own needs, and it has made me hopeful that

I can continue to perform, in creative ways, working with the parameters of illness.'

Marion echoes the sentiment while taking it further, expressing, via her computer, how vital it is for her emotional and mental wellbeing to embrace her creativity in whatever way remains possible to her. 'I've adapted my creativity umpteen times in line with what my body allows. So far, I've found a way. Making, writing and imagining feel as important as breathing. I don't think I could survive this stationary, isolated life of mine without. I can count the words I speak each day. Small mouthfuls in the morning, when energy is best. That's why writing is so important to me. I can push and pull sentences at my own slow pace, mull them over with eyes closed and they feel true and – hopefully – beautiful. My creations are emissaries, if you will, from bedland. I feel seen! My best spirits reside with my creative projects. Picking up the threads after worn-out days softens something in me that is in danger of calcifying.'

'Making, writing and imagining feel as important as breathing. My creations are emissaries from bedland.' - Marion

Karen has brought along her collage of overlapping scraps of maps, musical scores, book pages, word-searches and blank paper. These fragments are placed at different angles with hints of words, sentences, directions and broken paragraphs exposed. Some are only partially stuck down, fluttering up from the surface with other scraps stuck behind them. The effect draws you into its chaotic pattern. As we study her offering, she explains that in making it she was seeking 'to illustrate what brain fog is like. I was attempting to say something and it took four tries to get a simple sentence out.' There is a cohesion to the piece that works aesthetically while demonstrating confusion.

Ellie shares how knitting imparts its therapeutic rhythm on her days spent living with Hashimoto's disease and other health complications: 'I often reflect on how knitting has saved my sanity since I became ill, especially when I had to give up work. I have my needles to hand constantly; only at my sickest am I not able to pick them up. The warmth, colour and texture comfort, the metronomic clicking soothes, and I make things that matter. The way to express creativity sometimes has to be reinvented. I never knitted at all before I got sick. I can't write the way I could before, because of cognitive damage, and I think my prolific knitting output in part makes up for the difficulty with my writing.'

Andy is hand-stitching a sashiko pattern on patched-together scraps of fabric to make a boro cushion cover while musing, 'When the big things are removed from your life – a career, the ability to study, to drive, to walk, to interact with others in normal ways – only smallness is left. But in smallness there is beauty. Over 25 years of illness the small me met with other small parts of life and together we wove a small new world. I found haiku poems. I found knitting simple scarves and hats, traditional stitching patterns, and soft fabrics. Without illness I would have never discovered these things.'

Mary runs the online group Chronically Inspired. She observes that, 'In our creativity we inspire one another to persevere, to look beyond the pain, to adapt our art to our ever-changing needs, to transform the physical and emotional strain into something beautiful. When words cannot convey what we feel, art can fill that gap.' To the newest members of her group and this virtual circle we find ourselves in, she says, 'Just find one new hobby and try it out temporarily. You don't know where it will lead, who it will impact and how one small change will help you or someone else in the long run. You are still you, and you are still on your journey.'

The compassion and sense of relief at being among those who understand us in this circle are palpable. And it needn't remain only imagined. There are online groups as well as in-person gatherings that provide exactly what this imaginary scenario does.

Just knowing that there are others in similar situations to your own makes you an immediate member of a disparate group. If you haven't already, claim your virtual membership! We are all here, together at a distance.

Suggested creative exercise
Learning from another's path

Choose one of the artists mentioned in this chapter to investigate further. Alternatively, you may like to research other creators with health struggles. You will discover more throughout this book but in the meantime the poet **Emily Dickinson**, writer **Robert Louis Stevenson**, contemporary singer and musician **Ren**, and contemporary illustrator **Kyrianna Bolles** are a few leads to follow. Find out what you can about their chronic condition's impact on them. Absorb their creative output and consider what you like or dislike about it, what you might learn from it, and how you think it may have been different if they hadn't experienced chronic illness. Reflect on how you can relate this to your own health and creativity. Perhaps you'd like to consider Frida Kahlo's famous assertion that she painted because she had to and ask yourself what could become your creative saviour.

Artistic responses to illness at a glance

- Many famous artists of all genres have found their work to be influenced by their health.
- Not all ill health enhances creativity, but when encouraged to it can lead the artist in unexpected directions.
- As well as established professionals throughout history, there are numerous amateur artists and crafters who both use their health as inspiration for their art and use their art to help them navigate their health.

Part 2:

Creative healthcare

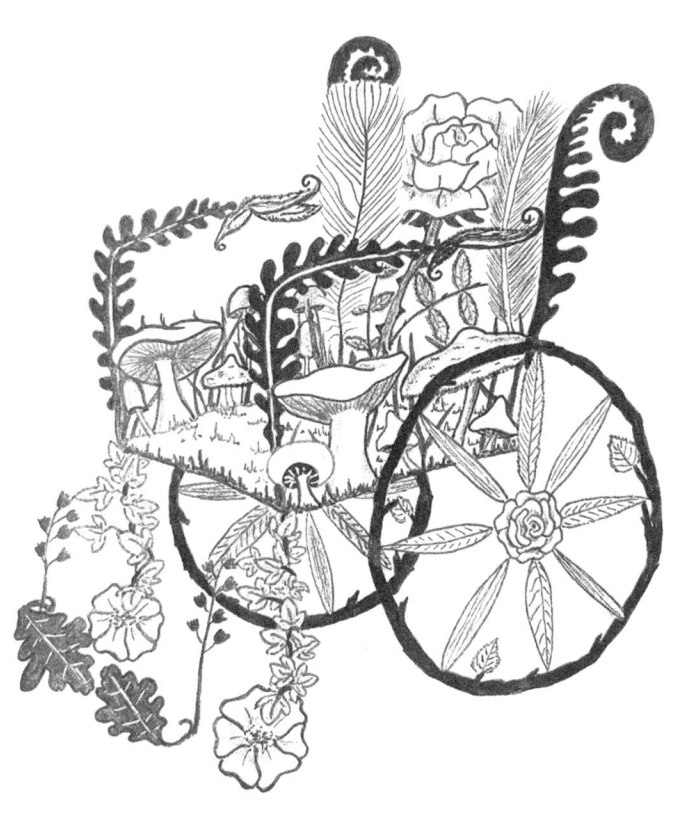

Chapter 4
An historical viewpoint

Arts and crafts have been used within medical and healing systems throughout the history of humanity. To learn more about the relationship between the arts and healing, let's embark on an educational time-travel adventure…

First stop: Ancient Greece

The concept of cathartic writing is familiar to many. It is used in therapeutic settings as a catalyst for emotional freedom and, sometimes, subsequent physical healing. This link between the arts and health dates to Ancient Greece when, in the fourth century BCE, Aristotle recognised the power of release not just through one's own writing but also via narratives written by others.

Nowadays, we differentiate between emotional catharsis and physical purging, but Aristotle used the term 'purging' to mean both medical and psychological catharsis. In his work *Poetics*, he stated that dramatic arts served as a 'purging of the spirit of morbid and base ideas or emotions by witnessing such emotions or ideas on stage'. That this was seen to bring about good health is demonstrated by the fact that a theatre was built for this very use in the grounds of a temple to Asclepius, the Greek god of medicine.

Temples to Asclepius were used as sites for theatrical performances, religious rites and communal contests. As well as hosting sporting events, they featured artistic contests in his honour. This association between medicine and the arts was later exemplified in the fifth century when the architects of the hospital halls of Athens designed them with the calming and curative effects of pleasing aesthetics in mind.

Music was also considered by Ancient Greeks as having healing powers. The Greek hero Odysseus was said to have been healed of his wounds not just by prosaic bandages, but also by the addition of chanting. By the eighth century BCE it was commonly thought that music could bring about pain relief and later, in *Politics*, Aristotle wrote of the effect music could have on listeners: 'All experience a certain purge and pleasant relief.' A few centuries later, Pythagoras was using a daily dose of singing to maintain good health, believing that it balanced the 'humours'.

Medicine and music across the continents and ages

It was in the third to first centuries BCE when the Ancient Chinese associated music with improved health, having made a link between the pentatonic (five-noted) musical scale and the five sensory organs of the human body. Music was thus used primarily as a healing tool and *The Yellow Emperor's Manual of Internal Medicine*, written at the time, details a doctor playing a bamboo pipe as medical treatment.

The strength with which music became linked to healing is demonstrated by the fact that the Chinese word for medicine – *yao* – when written in traditional Chinese character form combines the character for music with that for herbs.

Music was so highly regarded for its ability to sustain wellness that it became legally mandatory for students of medicine to also appreciate music.

Staying with the power of music but moving forwards in time and across to Europe, we can note that both the Roman statesman Cato and the philosopher Pliny wrote of incantations being used to aid the morale of patients being treated for a dislocated hip. This practice carried on into Mediaeval medicine, when alternating sounds of the flute and harp were used as a remedy for gout. In fact, during the Middle Ages, music was so highly regarded for its ability to sustain wellness that it became legally mandatory for students of medicine to also appreciate music.

Dr Kane, an early twentieth-century American surgeon, experimented with the effects of music and the spoken word being played on a phonograph in his operating room. An account published soon after, in the *American Yearbook of Anaesthesia and Analgesia*, records how it was the effect of the phonograph in recovery wards that inspired him to trial it in the operating theatre, leading to almost all of his patients better tolerating anaesthetic induction. This effect was also demonstrated in dentistry in the latter half of the twentieth century, when a combination of loud noises and background music brought about a decreased need for analgesia in patients undergoing painful procedures.

Arts and medicine in eleventh-century Perso-Arabia

In Persia, around 1025, a five-volume medical encyclopaedia, *The Canon of Medicine*, was compiled by Avicenna. He came to be considered the father of early modern medicine and continues to influence traditional Perso-Arabic medicine today. His work contains 150 mentions of the curative properties not only of music but of a selection of arts including dance, poetry, painting and sculpture.

Another eleventh century medical tome, *Maintenance of Health*, written by Ibn Butlan, an Arabian physician, was so well considered that it was translated into Latin in the thirteenth century. This treatise attends to the health benefits of the arts by drawing our attention to creative writing and oral storytelling. It proclaims that storytellers are 'one of the causes of sleep' as well as aiding 'digestion, senses and spirit'.

Art, religion and healing – from traditional cultures to modern day

From the First Nations of America to Siberian shamanic practice to medicine men and cunning women the world over, rhythmic chanting, drumming, dancing, retelling of mythologies and painted or crafted symbolic images are integrated into healing rites. They are not held apart as a luxury aesthetic but considered crucial to the wellbeing of the individual and their community, having both physical and esoteric relevance in the process of restoring health.

The definition of healing amongst indigenous cultures tends to encompass more than just physical sickness or injury and this isn't irrelevant to more modern societies. In 1978, the World Health Organization (WHO) defined holistic health as looking at the wholeness of a person within their wider environment, or words to that effect. In his book, *Illness and the Art of Creative Self-expression*, the paediatrician John Graham-Pole emphasises that even when the physical body is taken over by a chronic disability, a holistic interpretation of what constitutes healthiness is still available. The physical body is but one aspect of the whole person. This, along with a desire to seek supernatural assistance when our empirical knowledge doesn't yet possess the answers, is why healthcare the world over has often been affiliated with religious practice.

For a long time, Western healthcare was closely aligned with the church. Visual art in hospitals was of a religious nature to encourage patients to pray for healing. By the seventeenth century, filling hospitals with great works of art had become a philanthropic venture for the aristocracy and nobility. The more clinical approach to medicine in the early twentieth century saw a rapid decline in any use of artwork, religious iconography or pleasing aesthetics in medical settings, with colour and interior decoration becoming taboo in care environments.

Healthcare is about more than seeking cures or palliative care. It is an holistic process.

We have since returned to an understanding that the display of artwork in hospitals does have a beneficial effect, relieving anxiety, decreasing the perception of pain and enhancing emotional and physical recovery from medical procedures. We are perhaps coming full circle in our understanding that healthcare is about more than seeking cures or palliative care. It is an holistic process. In the interest of this, arts and creativity are being offered to patients not just in the sense of soaking up artists' creative offerings but as a pursuit to be actively involved in.

Chapter 4

The official emergence of art and craft therapy

In the nineteenth century, before effective medication was available, handcrafts such as basketry were considered a suitable activity for patients suffering from neurasthenia and psychiatric difficulties. However, it wasn't until the aftermath of the First and Second World Wars that crafting as occupational therapy and rehabilitation came into its own in Britain. Knitting, embroidery, woodwork, metalwork and, yes, basket weaving, were suggested to soldiers convalescing from physical wounds and suffering from what we would now call PTSD. The actor Ernest Thesiger, himself wounded by war, created sewing kits to be sent to injured soldiers to work on in their homes. This enterprise became known as the Disabled Soldiers' Embroidery Industry, with his own title being Honorary Secretary Cross-Stitch.

These diversional therapies were employed not just to distract soldiers from physical pain and negative ruminations but to rebuild wasted muscles, exercise hand-eye coordination and steady shaking hands. They were also designed to develop new skills that would help with re-entry into the civilian workplace.

The term 'art therapy' was coined in 1942 by Adrian Hill who practised it while convalescing from tuberculosis, and subsequently convinced the hospital authorities of its benefits. Art therapy developed into a health profession that has come to be considered predominantly useful in the field of mental health and emotional recovery. Back then, the Red Cross and the National Association for the Prevention of Tuberculosis were among the first agencies to employ it.

And back to the present day

Here in the twenty-first century, we are proud of the evidence-based bio-medical model and the scientific advances made in the world of medicine. Some of the more ancient beliefs about the connection between arts and healing have moved out of favour but they are by no means rejected by all. It is not only those who follow traditional routes to holistic wellness who appreciate these practices. More and more mainstream health professionals are espousing the power creative arts can have on physical, as well as mental and emotional, health.

While the Ancients provided theories that don't necessarily ring true for us now, perhaps they instinctively, and through practice, recognised the positive effects that engaging with the Arts could have on our minds and bodies, even if they hadn't yet worked out why. As we balance the desire to eradicate disease with an understanding that wellness includes living *well* with chronic afflictions, the recognition of arts, crafts and creativity as being relevant to those living with illness is once again coming to the fore, and it's not just patients who see the health value in creative pursuits.

Ancient peoples recognised the positive effects that engaging with the arts could have on our minds and bodies, even if they hadn't yet worked out why.

In a paper on arts, health and wellbeing, the Welsh NHS Confederation affirms that engaging with Arts in addition to medical care can not only improve mental health but physical wellbeing, too. Many GPs now follow the practice of social prescribing, which directs patients to social networks, including gardening clubs, art and craft groups, and choirs. In the next two chapters we'll find out more about how these may be specifically beneficial to physical and emotional health.

Suggested therapeutic activity

A medical incantation

The chants and incantations that Ancients employed alongside their medical treatments may have had a beneficial effect by encouraging certain actions or taking a relevant length of time to recite, much like the instruction to sing *Happy Birthday* while washing hands during the COVID-19 pandemic. With this in mind, create a rhyme, song or verbal charm that can assist your health routine in some way. Perhaps the words will remind you when to take different medications, or the duration may guide you in how long to hold remedial stretches for. It could be a rhythmic reminder of a beneficial state of mind or behaviour, a soothing song to occupy you when symptoms are difficult, or a whimsical ditty that makes tedious treatments pass more quickly. Witty or mystical, it's your incantation so go in whatever direction suits you.

An historical viewpoint at a glance

- There are different types of wellbeing – from physical, to emotional, to spiritual.
- Throughout history and around the world, arts and crafts have been employed across this wide genre of healthcare.
- Cathartic theatre, music, storytelling, symbolic images and visual arts have all been documented throughout history as being used to promote good health.
- While art therapy has primarily been seen in the West as a tool for fixing the psyche, it has also been recognised as having legitimate effects on the physical body.

Chapter 5
Crafty prescriptions for physical conditions

Hospitals, support groups, clinical studies and people in their homes have repeatedly found arts and crafts to be beneficial to those with physical health problems. It is widely accepted that engaging with visual arts, musical arts and expressive writing (both as an active participant and as an appreciator of others' work) can reduce stress levels. Less well known is that they have been demonstrated to have a positive impact on patients' vital functions, nutrient levels, immune function, motor skills, mental agility, physical pain, insomnia and depression.

First, let's consider how creativity in general impacts the brain before we look at the specific effects of different creative practices.

Arts and neuroplasticity

Neuroplasticity is the brain and nervous system's ability to change through exposure to experience. It is enhanced by practising any new skill, and many people use foreign languages, crosswords, sudokus, or strategic games like chess, to maintain their brain health. However, it turns out that engaging in any creative activity, including cookery or reading other people's creative works, can have a similar effect on cognitive strength. Arts and crafts, it would seem, can structurally change your brain.

Arts and crafts can structurally change your brain.

The areas in the brain needed for maintaining concentration, planning, memory, spatial awareness, sensory input, precision of motor skills and timing of movement are all activated through engagement with various creative pursuits. Practising a gently challenging craft, while utilising as many senses as possible, simultaneously relaxes the nervous system while strengthening these different departments and the connections between them. By doing this we may be able to mitigate some of the cognitive impairment that can accompany chronic health conditions. A 2012 study, held at the Mayo Clinic, lends weight to this hope. It found that if people with early-stage age-related dementia and cognitive impairment participated in activities such as knitting, quilting, reading and game-playing, they were 30-50% less likely to have mild cognitive impairment than those who didn't take part in these activities.

There are so many skills and techniques to be discovered within the varied world of arts and crafts that it is an almost limitless way of keeping your brain as responsive and healthy as possible.

The one downside of this is that learning new skills can be hard work for those with existing cognitive impairment. However, we can work with this by beginning with a very simple craft and being gentle with our expectations. Don't put pressure on yourself to uncover your inner craft genius or master artist if you want the full therapeutic value. For the best effect, you want to both relax and very gently exercise your brain and body. Keep practising your starter skill until experience kicks in, and you expend less energy performing it, before moving on to the next stage. Procedural memory will gradually ensure that the various stages come more naturally, and you may soon be wondering what you found so difficult.

Doodling, drawing, colouring and sculpting

An endeavour that requires no practice or learned technique is the art of doodling. Girija Kaimal, author of *The Expressive Instinct – How Imagination and Creative Works Help Us Survive and Thrive*, tells us that doodling is an undervalued tool for improving memory. Drawing and sculpting can also activate memory processes and spatial-temporal processing, thanks to their effects on gamma and theta power in specific parts of the brain.

Along with drawing, sculpting and colouring, doodling increases blood flow to the pre-fontal cortex, potentially igniting pleasurable feelings of reward, so how about colouring in your doodles? The effects of colouring can be further enhanced by choosing to colour mandalas while sitting outside in nature. Doing so has been shown to lower cortisol levels and pain intensity. If getting outside isn't an option, then houseplants and flowers indoors may replicate the effect.

Textile crafts

Yarn crafts have seen a resurgence in popularity over recent years. As such, it is probably to be expected that much of the research on the therapeutic benefits of crafting have focused on knitting and crochet.

A study carried out by the *British Journal of Occupational Therapy* noted that those who were more frequent knitters reported better cognitive abilities than those who didn't knit so often. Meanwhile, the charity Knit for Peace commissioned an evidence-based study on the mental and physical health benefits of knitting. Their conclusion was that the act of knitting can delay the onset of dementia, ease depression and function as a distraction from chronic pain. Specifically, they learnt from one survey that 92% of the participants who reported being in very poor health felt knitting had a beneficial effect on their health and improved their mood, while 82% said they found it relaxing.

Studies have also shown that knitting and crochet can lower blood pressure. The comedian Jenny Eclair noted this recognised physical benefit when she recalled being advised to take up knitting to help combat the high blood pressure she was experiencing during perimenopause. The health benefits of knitting and crochet generally focus on the relaxing action of rhythmic movement as well as being beneficial for conditions that require gentle exercise to keep joints supple. As such, embroidery, cross-stitch and all types of needlework, as well as many other textile or mixed media crafts, lend themselves to this outcome.

Engaging in textile arts has also been shown to encourage the lowering of inflammatory markers released by the immune system, thus potentially reducing inflammatory symptom flares in the body.

Writing

Creative writing has long been utilised by art therapists, counsellors and individuals as a cathartic act. Releasing emotions that have no other safe channel in which to be directed is good medicine, helping to lighten the load of stress the body is carrying. Indeed, expressive writing has been demonstrated to increase heart rate variability – a sign that the heart is responding better to stress – and to lower elevated blood pressure.

Listening to poetry can reduce pain intensity as well as helping combat insomnia.

Practised regularly, creative writing can help alleviate depressive feelings, which in turn can put one in a mental space better equipped to follow medical advice and health regimes. Even just listening to poetry can reduce pain intensity as well as helping combat insomnia when enjoyed at bedtime.

More surprisingly, a study with HIV patients showed that 30 minutes a day of expressive writing for four days resulted in a drop in viral load. This suggests a particularly strong link between stress levels and our immune function. The effect may not be maintained over time and could be influenced by how freely patients already consciously express themselves. Nevertheless, it is a worthwhile tool to have in the chronically ill person's creative supply box.

Chapter 5

Music and gardening

It is well known that learning a musical instrument at a young age can enhance cognitive abilities and encourage continued neuroplasticity. What many don't realise is that playing an instrument at any age helps the brain to continue nurturing these connections. Further to this, just listening to music can have a beneficial effect.

Classical music, especially, is recommended for combating high blood pressure and muscle tension, and it has been shown that the grey matter of the brain in people who have had strokes is changed for the better by listening to music. Anecdotal evidence that the brain waves of severe ME patients show similarities to those of stroke patients further suggests the benefits music could potentially bestow.

In fact, exposure to rhythmic music has been seen to have a notable positive effect on a variety of conditions including MS, COPD, brain trauma, Parkinson's disease, Huntingdon's disease and spinal cord injuries. According to Dr John Graham-Pole, music can aid recovery from heart attacks, speed up growth and development in newborn babies, stimulate mental clarity, improve tolerance to painful treatments and reduce attention to painful symptoms. Separate research also suggests auditory stimulation can reduce pain, especially for cancer patients and people requiring anaesthesia.

An experiment conducted at University College London with a group of critically ill patients showed that exposure to Mozart's music caused growth hormone plasma concentrations to increase significantly and stress response hormones to drop, which resulted, to a degree, in the immune system being regulated. And at least two studies (one focusing on post-operative nausea, the other on patients undergoing chemotherapy) have shown that listening to music can reduce nausea and vomiting. Music is also believed to speed up slow gastric motility and therefore enhance digestion.

Physiotherapy to improve standing and walking is enhanced when music is playing, and mindful-based dance movement therapy has been shown to lessen pain levels of chronic headache sufferers. In conditions that require you to push yourself to increase motility, music is beneficial in its ability to encourage more physical movement. However, I mention this with the caveat to always take care to stay within your own safe limits. Some chronic illnesses are worsened by movement or energy use. In these cases, music can have a stimulating effect that may increase symptoms. Due to hyperacuity making me sensitive to sounds and my heart rate being raised by musical beats, the music I most enjoy can leave me feeling dizzy, nauseated and physically exhausted. In contrast, careful choice of classical piano or cello music, peaceful flute compositions, or pieces composed for relaxation have a calming effect.

These examples clearly demonstrate that you don't need to be able to make your own music. Enjoying other people's creative output can be just as positive for those living with severe conditions. If, however, you'd rather be an active participant, you may like to know that singing and playing some wind and brass instruments can increase lung function and breath control. Meanwhile, multiple studies have demonstrated that humming may help keep sinuses clear and healthy. Humming is also thought to stimulate and tone the vagus nerve, which can have a positive effect on an over-reactive stress response in the body and conditions such as postural tachycardia syndrome (PoTS).

> *The balance and harmony that we respond to in music are also present in natural forms such as flower displays.*

The neurologist Oliver Sacks noted that the balance and harmony that we respond to in music are also present in natural forms such as flower displays, however elaborate or simple they may be. Our brains find this sensory input a calming and naturally organising influence. For this reason, he cited gardens and music as being valuable non-pharmaceutical therapies in chronic neurological illness. Gazing at plants provides gentler stimulation for the brain than looking at most manmade architecture or objects. Fractal patterning, often occurring in nature, is a design in which the pattern is repeated endlessly in different sizes. Because of this inbuilt predictability, the human brain can relax and the eyes make fewer movements when gazing at such objects as Romanesco broccoli, pinecones, leaf veins or vistas like river deltas that contain fractal patterns.

Gardening (described as landscape painting by the poet Alexander Pope), depicting and photographing plants, or arranging cut or living flowers, all unite personal creativity with the natural world.

Suggested therapeutic activity
Express yourself

Choose a blank-paged book that you will enjoy using and give yourself permission to fill it freely. This book is not to be saved for best. It is your creative expression diary. In it you can write your darkest feelings, brightest hopes and strangest dreams. Doodle, draw patterns to colour in, jot down interesting words, record half-formed ideas, create verse, sketch what you see, stick things in, cut out shapes, and turn the pages into an extension of you.

A range of pencils from soft to hard, coloured pencils or crayons, a favoured writing pen, and a couple of different thickness fine-liner pens will help you vary the way you express yourself on the page. You may also want to gather old magazines and papers for collaging. If so, a pair of scissors and a basic glue stick will come in handy, too.

When stuck for ideas, start with an observation of something you can see, hear, smell or feel and see where this leads you, emotionally. You might also find it interesting to sing or hum to yourself, either just before or while working on your diary. Notice whether your choice of music affects what arrives on the page.

Crafty prescriptions for physical conditions at a glance

- Learning new skills and practising crafts can combat cognitive impairment.
- Creative expression as simple as doodling has beneficial effects on the brain.
- Knitting, crochet and sewing have multiple benefits for health, including distraction from pain, lowered blood pressure and reduction of inflammatory markers.
- Expressive writing can increase heart rate variability and have positive effects on the immune system.
- Passive and interactive exposure to music has a positive effect on many conditions.
- Fractal patterns (commonly found in nature) and gardens are potentially good therapy for neurological conditions.

Chapter 6
Creative calm for happier health

To state that less stress equals better health is not to say that illness will be cured by a positive approach, the correct thoughts, or a charmed life. Chronic illness is most frequently physical in origin (even sometimes when presenting as a mental health condition), often highly debilitating, and not the fault of the person living with it. That said, it is undeniable that stress puts a strain on the body, especially one working extra hard to maintain functionality. The cardiovascular, endocrine, gastrointestinal, musculoskeletal, nervous, reproductive and respiratory systems are all known to be influenced by stress levels, so it would be remiss not to look at how stress can affect our health conditions.

Learning a little about the HPA (hypothalamus–pituitary–adrenal) axis taught me a lot about how my chronically ill body responds to stress, including the positive stress of being excited about something or laughing exuberantly. To sum up: when the body perceives stress of any kind (physical, chemical, nutritional, mental, emotional), changes take place in the body. Bodies that are already under existing pressure to cope with an acquired or in-born condition are primed to be on high alert. The HPA axis is ever ready and raring to react. This can activate the sympathetic nervous system (going into fight or flight mode, as far as you and I are concerned), either at a subtle or super-enhanced level, and the body releases hormones that instruct muscles, mind, gut, immune system and more to behave in ways that are often only helpful if you need to run or attack. The result? Exacerbation of existing symptoms as well as a whole gamut of new ones for some.

So, a calm life, sedate hobbies and an array of relaxation techniques become our arsenal against any influence threatening to aggravate our sympathetic nervous system. This isn't just about finding relaxing distractions to help us cope with our condition, although that is particularly valid. It is about encouraging the body into as calm, un-alarmed, and stable a state as possible, before symptoms flare. And it turns out that arts and crafts are perfect candidates for the job.

Enjoying arts and crafts has been found to positively affect the amygdala, hippocampus and medial orbitofrontal cortex of the brain, all of which are critical to a balanced stress response, feelings of reward, and emotional processing. As such, this genre of activities helps to alleviate emotional distress, anxiety and depression while enhancing communication skills, involvement in the community and a sense of self-identity – all aspects of life that can be dented by long-term ill health.

Whether we are consciously aware of it or not, embarking on a creative project can provide a calm yet focused reason to carry on with another day of illness. It becomes material proof of our existence when we feel we are disappearing behind the cloak of illness. Engaging in a craft is what reminds some that their life still has reason. It is both a practical and a constructive activity as other interests are necessarily set aside. The metaphoric importance of arts and crafts that piece different elements together to create something whole is important, too. Patchwork, collaging and upcycling are all examples of crafts that boost a sense of resurrection and substance when the rest of our life feels diminished or torn apart.

Embarking on a creative project can provide a calm yet focused reason to carry on with another day of illness.

It is no wonder then that, according to a study conducted by researchers at Drexel University in 2016, 45 minutes of creative art, regardless of skill level, significantly lowers cortisol levels in the body. With this stress-related hormone under control, it's not just the more noticeable symptoms of the fight or flight response that are soothed away. When we are stressed, our gut's microbiome becomes altered, which in turn influences the regulation of neurotransmitters in the brain. A scientific paper somewhat cumbersomely entitled, 'The effects of stress and meditation on the immune system, human microbiota, and epigenetics', concluded that when we attain a calm state, helped along by meditation, the balance in our gut is restored. This, in turn, calms inflammation and encourages healthier gut-barrier function. 'But that paper was about meditation, not crafts,' you may say. ('And meditation is boring,' a few of you may mutter under your breath.) I hear you, and I have good news for any meditation-averse crafters.

A crafty approach to meditation

No matter how much you recognise the benefits of a zen-like mindset, if your health requires you to be immobile much of the time you may find yourself craving movement and resisting motionless meditation. While some people prefer yoga, tai chi or walking meditations to sitting or lying still, those of us unable to partake in more energy-intensive movements can rejoice in the fact that repetitive simple crafts have their own meditative effect.

The gentle focus and rhythmic movements of a craft that doesn't strain your physical or cognitive abilities can generate a sense of calm in both mind and body. Many crafters find the clicking of knitting needles, or the sound of thread drawing through cloth pulled taut on an embroidery hoop, has a soothing, almost hypnotic, effect. Choose your tools and materials accordingly to gain maximum benefit. Some love the warm texture and soft sound of bamboo knitting needles whereas I find the cool touch and traditional click of my Nanna's metal knitting needles more pleasing. Giving our senses something pleasurably familiar to settle on when feeling agitated, frustrated, consumed with pain or wired with overtiredness can encourage our whole system to relax into a more meditative and healthy state.

Practising your creative hobby can also replicate meditation by encouraging you to hold your attention in the current moment rather than ruminating on the past or future. The present can be a difficult place to entrust yourself to when plagued by physical pain or mental distress, so this is where crafts come into their own. They provide an opportunity to focus on a gently pleasant stimulus that exists in the now but outside of your suffering. Through this creative distraction, the forefront of your mind receives a little respite from focusing on the trials of the body while also benefiting from the pain-relieving chemicals released in the brain. This can be a space, if only for a few moments, to relax away from any bigger concerns than where next to place your sewing needle or what colour pencil to choose.

You may decide to deepen the meditative effect by placing your attention solely on the counting of stitches or reciting a mnemonic rhyme for the movements of your craft, as a mantra. Or you might prefer to experiment with meditative creations through paying attention to your senses, allowing your awareness to rest on the tapping of computer keys or the slap of paint and drag of brush on canvas. Perhaps you resonate best with colour and enjoy letting your eyes absorb the hues you've chosen to work with, reflecting on how they make you feel and imagining yourself inhaling the colours as you work? Choose any of your senses and let your mind explore the full experience of your chosen craft.

In Tibetan Buddhism, intricately patterned mandalas are created over months from coloured sand before being swept entirely away. This creative form of ritualistic destruction is performed as a meditation on the impermanence of all experience. In an extension of this practice, we can produce items designed to decompose, be cleared away or consumed, regarding our creativity as a valued moment in time. We are free to breathe it out, let it go; tear it up, unravel or delete it.

Transient creations help us to be on better terms with the ephemeral nature of our health. Good times may feel brief and blow away easily, but weighty emotions also lift and give way to new. Whether or not we choose to symbolically align our creative actions with feelings about our health, we are priming ourselves to be reminded that, however constant our condition feels, the strength of symptoms and occurrence of relapses rise and fall. All is transitory. We are not in a fixed state of suffering. Neither should we expect unfaltering contentment. There is a calmness that settles when we accept the universality of this.

Anxiety and depression

Whether anxiety and depression are key clinical symptoms for you or side-effects of coping day-and-night in, day-and-night out, with a misbehaving body, there's no denying that physical and mental health conditions are often enforced companions. So, it's worth knowing that the repetitive and often rhythmic hand movements required in crafting can trigger the release of serotonin, dopamine and other feel-good chemicals in the brain that influence hormonal secretions to precipitate a calmer state of being.

A study on knitting entitled, 'The benefits of knitting for personal and social wellbeing in adulthood: Findings from an international survey', found that the more frequently the participants knitted, the more calm and happy they felt. Their research deduced that knitting and crochet not only distract from pain and provide

Rhythmic hand movements required in crafting can trigger the release of serotonin, dopamine and other feel-good chemicals in the brain.

a relaxing opportunity to express creativity (especially at times of reduced physical capacity), but also reduce depression and anxiety. A small 2009 study on how knitting affected women hospitalised with anorexia, demonstrated that knitting for an average of one hour and 20 minutes a day for a few weeks resulted in 74% feeling less anxious or preoccupied by their condition.

The combination of occupying your hands while directing your attention towards a specific, achievable task particularly helps to channel the nervous energy of agitation that can come with anxiety. Jittery fingers and negative thoughts are steered away from urges to self-harm as an alternative focus is provided. Concentration levels, impacted by anxiety and depression, often find that simple projects prove the most effective remedy. Even those who don't generally suffer from anxiety can benefit from the calming effects of rhythmic crafts, such as crochet, cross-stitch or knitting, when waiting for medical appointments or anticipating test results. Selina, who, like many chronically ill patients, has concerns about how she will be treated by the medical establishment, certainly finds this the case. 'I'm so thankful for crafting,' she says. 'It gives me an anchor to focus on and to hold me down when I'm facing something like seeing the consultant.'

According to Sue Stuart-Smith, in her book *The Well Gardened Mind*, being in a garden or having flowering plants within sight, increases alpha waves in the brain. This, in turn, releases serotonin along with its calming and mood-uplifting benefits. Whether you choose to embroider, paint, photograph, arrange or grow plants, a natural subject matter for visual arts and crafts offers added benefits.

But don't worry if working with visual arts or gardening isn't your thing. Dr John Graham-Pole maintains that music improves the lives of patients with long-term (and terminal) illness by reducing anxiety. Both listening to and playing music can have calming effects on neural activity in the brain, which in turn affects the hypothalamus and amygdala (remember that HPA axis?), calming the nervous systems, including heart rate, breathing and digestion.

When choosing what to listen to or play, the most important factor is what appeals to you and how it makes you feel, but it's worth bearing in mind that slow music written in the key of C major, A major or E flat major can have a particularly peaceful, calming effect. Alpha brain waves (the waves associated with relaxation) synchronise with music played at 60 beats per minute, while delta brain waves (those involved with falling asleep) will attune to even slower music, so select your tunes in accordance with your desired result. When suffering with cortisol and adrenaline imbalances that resulted in extreme levels of physical agitation, a racing and pounding heart, twitching, shaking and a sensation of abject terror, playing the piano has given me moments of enough respite to recoup some strength for the next onslaught of symptoms. I found the act of engaging both my mind and fingers on playing a piece that I was familiar with enabled me to move very slightly beyond what my body was experiencing into a space that soothed me just enough to feel I could cope. My favourite genres of piano music to play are jazz and blues, but the piece that soothes me the most when in the throes of a severe adrenaline attack is Bach's *Well Tempered Clavichord* – a gently flowing and relatively easy-to-play piece.

Re-directing difficult emotions

Being home alone with pain, boredom, depression or anxiety is an open invitation to coping mechanisms such as comfort eating, smoking, drinking, nail biting, self-harm or mindless online scrolling. Engaging our hands and mind with creative hobbies of any genre is an enjoyable way to stave off destructive responses that could otherwise creep through our days. We can embrace this further by specifically choosing crafts that exorcise unhelpful urges and support our mental health. For example, when severe adrenaline surges were putting agitated images of cutting myself in my mind, I decided to use that destructive energy to tear blades of grass from the ground and use these in an art piece. Plucking the leaves with force felt therapeutic, while consciously deciding to replace the image of knife blades with blades of grass helped me to process my feelings constructively.

There are many creative techniques that you might find beneficial when consumed with dark feelings, intrusive impulses or negative thoughts. When a sense of calm is out of immediate reach, motions that absorb the urge to physically react to stress are the next best step. Needle felting requires you to repeatedly stab the wool. Smashing up unloved or broken crockery to reassemble as a mosaic is both therapeutic and a powerfully symbolic act. Paper cutting is a satisfying use of an actual blade, but if this doesn't feel a safe option for you then torn paper creations (including collages made from old photographs, postcards, maps or discarded art) can be very effective. Write or draw or sing excess tension out of your system. Beat butter and sugar together until they wouldn't dare not rise for any ingredients they're baked with. Your use of colour may additionally embrace the feelings within, letting this aspect of you feel acknowledged and accepted, perhaps drawing it out of you.

If moving away from overwhelming feelings seems a more constructive approach for you, then choose a craft that generates a relaxed rhythm; one that even a mind struggling to concentrate can focus on rather than wandering into dark territory. Sing or hum to your plants as you artfully tend to them. Pick materials with textures that are comforting to touch, choose colours that uplift or soothe you, and take your time. Slow stitching is a trend that embraces leisurely hand stitching over sewing machines or a desire to attain speedy completion, and embraces knitting and crochet as well as sewing. Enjoy long exhales that reflect the gentle tempo. Deep out-breaths and sighs are one of your body's ways of lowering its heart rate and relaxing an anxious state, as well as improving lung function.

Alleviating trauma

It is becoming accepted that trauma can sometimes lodge in the body, manifesting as ailments if left undealt with. There is also greater awareness now around medical trauma. This is where the illness itself isn't caused by a distressing incident but, in fact, the reverse. Invasive procedures, lack of adequate healthcare, disbelief about one's symptoms, inappropriate behaviour from healthcare workers, insufficient support, and extreme health problems themselves can all lead to medical trauma. Living with chronic illness is challenging enough without added layers of suffering that further disrupt our equilibrium.

By making art that represents your illness or traumatic health memories, you give yourself an opportunity to work through your feelings at a slight remove. Through handling the tools of your creativity with this chosen focus, you learn to handle your experience, to process it and, when your creation is complete, set it aside. The artwork can, to a degree, contain it for you.

In the 1980s Francine Shapiro, an American psychotherapist, discovered that moving her eyes from left to right as she walked and let her mind focus on troublesome thoughts alleviated her distress. She developed this technique, including constructive reframing of thoughts under the guidance of a therapist, into a treatment known as Eye Movement Desensitisation and Reprocessing (EMDR). EMDR is now offered to sufferers of PTSD, phobias, anxiety and the stress that can accompany cancer and other physical conditions. The suggestion has since been made that any bilateral movement (not just of the eyes) could be of similar benefit. Walking and general exercise are obvious suggestions but, for those of us with limited mobility, arts and crafts that use both hands, although not a substitute for professional therapy, could be helpful. Employing both hands, we can muse on replacing traumatic responses or a negative mindset with more calmly constructive ones.

Making art that represents your illness or traumatic health memories, you give yourself an opportunity to work through your feelings at a slight remove.

Bilateral movement or otherwise, any form of creative art has the potential to bring relief. By putting personal experiences and emotions into our creations and then stepping back, we afford ourselves a little distance from our pain-generated reactions. This may enable us to consider our situation with some freedom from charged emotions, opening a gateway to more relaxed and helpful perceptions.

Grief and loss are recognised as having the potential to traumatise and yet how many of us cope with the daily loss of who we used to be, the life we used to engage in, or the future we had hoped for ourselves, without acknowledging that this is indeed a form of grief? Creative expression can help with processing these recurring feelings, but what about when our grief is for the loss of our artistic identity? It's worth recalling the adage that grief is love with nowhere to go. With that in mind, how could our love for a previous activity be re-directed? Sue Duda, now a batik artist but once a potter, has rheumatoid arthritis. She learned to adapt her creativity to suit her body's needs so that her loss could be channelled into a new pathway. 'Drawing was easier on my back, wrists and hands than my work as a stoneware potter. Although I grieved the loss of my identity as a potter, eventually I realized I did not have to give up being creative. I just needed to be creative in a different way. Drawing enabled me to experience the cheerfulness of color, without pain.'

Illness cognition

'Illness cognition' refers to a person's need to redefine their identity when they become ill. There is so much to adjust to when chronic illness takes centre stage. Daily limitations and physical requirements, loss or reduction of working life, the new dynamics within relationships, having to accept regular help and a reduced social life, all take their toll on how we perceive ourselves. Aspects of our previous existence and of future dreams are burnt away by disease, and some of the landmarks we navigated by fade into the fog of illness. When this happens, art can help us regain our bearings. It can assist us in maintaining our expression of our deeper nature or in reconstructing a newly appropriate personal identity, as we saw with Sue Duda.

Even if you've carried chronic illness your whole life, you will probably find you have expectations and visions for yourself based on the healthy lives around you. Settling comfortably into an identity that acknowledges your limitations and serves your needs while still allowing you to feel enjoyably alive and invigorated can be a long process.

For many ill or disabled people in our predominantly able-bodied, achievement-driven society, it is all too easy to label oneself a faulty anomaly. Being seen (or assuming we are seen) as just a medical patient – a disabled, dependent, quiet person who stays at home – is intensely frustrating when there are passions and ideas, exuberance and life choices all dancing inside, desperate to spiral outwards and break free. We can use art projects to convey who we'd like to be, were we not limited by illness, and to communicate how we'd like others to see us. This in turn feeds back into our own perception, nurturing a positive self-image.

Sam is a perfect example of this. A couple of years after being diagnosed with a disabling brain injury he decided to create a patchwork quilt. His idea was for each square to be a textile depiction of something he was still able to do despite the bodily limitations he was coming to terms with. His first square featured appliqué and embroidery detailing his love of dance. Even though he now suffers afterwards for very short dance sessions with his children, adding this square to his project reminded him that he hadn't entirely lost his old self. It was a celebration of who he still is. A poem he wrote to accompany this textile square also recognised the metaphorical way he can still welcome dance into the story of his days: 'I am Dance Able/I am able to move to the unanticipated rhythms of my life.'

The personal agency and strength of character that Sam's creative offerings present are a vibrant contrast to more traditional portrayals of ill health. In her book, *Portrait Therapy*, Susan M D Carr observes that if we look at historical portraits of illness, we usually see either an objectified representation of the ill person (Luis Jiménez Aranda's celebrated nineteenth century oil painting 'A Hospital Ward During the Chief Physician's Round' being one example) or a romanticised idea of them (as in 19th century portraits, such as Dante Gabriel Rossetti's depictions of Elizabeth Siddal, that glorified the pale, delicate appearance of consumptive patients), but not their individual selfhood. By portraying our lived experience as we wish to represent it, we exercise our voice of individuality and self-advocacy. The knock-on effect of this is a strengthened sense of self beyond the limitations of our health.

> *By portraying our lived experience as we wish to represent it, we exercise our voice of individuality and self-advocacy.*

Feeling this within ourselves, as well as having it better recognised by others, results in less stressful encounters and greater mental and physical equilibrium.

Creating confidence and resilience

Creativity leads the way to discovering an autonomy and ability that our body might seem to have stripped us of. Through art, we can turn an unchosen and unpleasant circumstance into something constructive, perhaps even beautiful. This is power: not power over the illness but a calm power within it. We are collaborating with our body.

When elements of our health conspire to change the way we view and express ourselves, this becomes especially important. We may have previously been known as confident, capable, lively and enthusiastic. We may still feel these attributes at the core of our personality, beneath the sludge of symptoms, but illness forces us to withdraw – and if we weren't of an outgoing nature before, long-term illness has a habit of compounding shyness and low self-esteem. Running on reduced energy and increased risk has a habit of sloughing away confidence. One way to combat this and re-develop some of that self-confidence is through a new skill that we can feel in charge of. Emma, who lives with chronic health conditions, has found this to be true. She notes that, 'I've struggled with confidence for a long time … but weaving is like therapy for me. It's given me so many insights above and over what I've learned about myself through therapy sessions.'

A sense of overwhelm when confronted with our symptoms can lead us to focus on what we can't do rather than what we can. Giving ourselves dedicated space and time to immerse in an endeavour we not only enjoy but can exert some control over, is an important routine to adopt. No longer need we feel entirely at the whims of our condition. The implicit confidence that this generates can instil a greater sense of calm in the face of the stresses that chronic illness so often delivers.

Becoming adept at an initially tricky craft demonstrates our capability to learn new strategies and techniques. We are teaching our brain that we do indeed have agency. Remaining calm in the face of generalised stress becomes easier with this knowledge. When we see that we can affect outcomes, be that merely the mark a pencil makes on paper or the transformation of a ball of yarn into a useable item, our self-belief spreads further. By discovering that solutions, new perspectives, progress and small successes are available to us, we learn to trust in our resilience and feel safer wherever we find ourselves.

With more examples of our creative and dexterous development, we absorb an assumption of our ability to rebound from setbacks, find solutions and generally build a resilient response to difficulties. There then becomes a greater likelihood of us engaging calmly and willingly in healthy behaviour such as setting boundaries or engaging with appropriate medical advice and self-care.

We may even discover that by appreciating our own creative output we are able to see ourselves afresh. Feeling proud of what we have made is one step closer to feeling more confident in general. Could this then generate the compassion or admiration we would naturally bestow on someone else in our situation but perhaps hadn't offered ourselves? If so, we will be gifting ourselves with a calmer overview of ourselves.

Suggested therapeutic activity
Colour wash

Most of us have experienced how different colours can affect our mood. Take a moment now to sit or lie comfortably and consider what colour would help you to relax or feel better. Imagine a wash of this colour flowing over and through you, or a diaphanous drape of coloured chiffon landing gently on and around you, permeating your being. If you require a more solid sensation, wrap yourself in an imaginary blanket of your chosen colour.

This exercise can be especially beneficial when experiencing emotional discomfort or physical symptoms that are eliciting difficult emotions. Ask yourself what colour represents your discomfort. If you have trouble ascribing it a colour, consider what other descriptive words might help you. Is the pain bruised, burning, fizzy, dull? These adjectives may generate associated colours for you. Imagine water diluting the original depth of colour. You could also apply white to it with an imagined soft brush and then introduce fresh colour.

If you feel able, choose a repetitive, absorbing craft (drawing, hand sewing, crochet, colouring, painting, the cutting and sticking of collaging, etc.) to use the colours you felt drawn to in this exercise. How can your craft celebrate the parts of your body that work well and bring compassion to those that don't?

Creative calm for better health at a glance

- Physical conditions are often exacerbated by stress.
- Creative arts, at any skill level, reduce stress hormones.
- The repetitive movements of some arts and crafts, combined with focused attention, have a meditative effect that can aid relaxation and ease some symptoms.
- Disposable art can be freeing and remind us that nothing is forever.
- Slow music has the most peaceful effect on the brain.
- Creative hobbies are a positive replacement for less constructive coping habits. The type of craft you choose can be cathartic or comforting, depending on your needs.
- Creative expression helps us to process medical trauma, stress, grief and other emotions surrounding long-term conditions. Hobbies that use both the left and right hands may alleviate stuck trauma.
- Art can be used to nurture a new, strengthened identity when our old self feels depleted.
- Becoming adept at a craft encourages confidence and resilience in the face of circumstances beyond our control.

Part 3:

The art of feeling larger than your illness

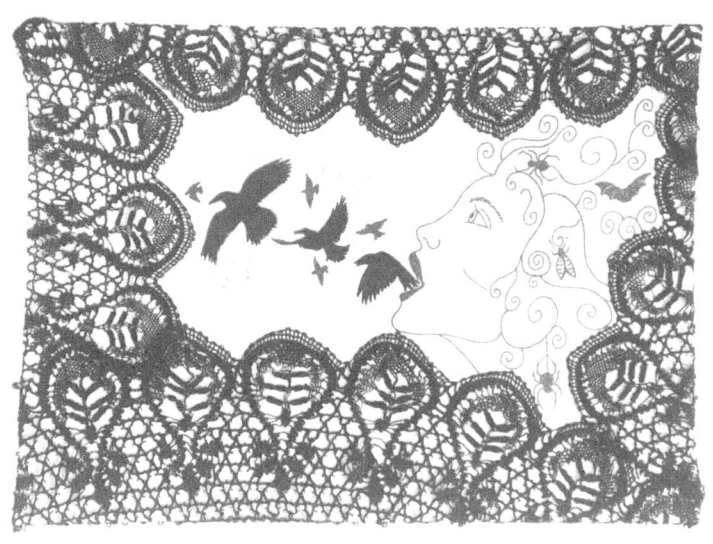

Chapter 7
Creating purpose

I used to struggle with finding a sense of purpose. I have been unwell since childhood and, although a brief time of stronger health combined with large doses of denial had resulted in my having a child, I rapidly became too unwell to look after her. I hadn't managed further education, begun a career or fulfilled my expectations of parenthood. I wasn't well enough to enter a workforce, or for a long while to volunteer any services, and was limited in my friendships. What did I contribute to society? What was the point of my existence?

Purpose: A predictor of healthy survival

This isn't the place for an existential discussion about the value of our lives. It is, however, important to recognise that the need to uncover a sense of purpose has effects on our physical as well as mental health. Studies have found lower rates of heart attacks, stroke and Alzheimer's disease, slower development of cognitive decline, fewer psychologically triggered symptoms and faster recovery from certain types of surgery in those with a personal sense of purpose. Feeling purposeful can impact our overall sense of wellbeing and how our physical condition affects us.

What brings meaning to your life will be entirely individual. It isn't important what area of life you find it in. What matters is that it is there and that you recognise it. Do you feel your life has a constructive focus or that your daily activities are engaging, important? While some people have a clear understanding, which flows in a steady direction, of what they are here to do, for many of us purpose is flexible. It changes with time and circumstance and may not even be something we pay much attention to when life is rolling busily along its regular route. But when the expected avenues are closed off, we find ourselves in search of alternative ways to express the values and experiences that hold meaning for us.

A day without visitors or outings; months without social get-togethers or being able to independently care for ourselves, let alone others; years without study, a career or holidays to look forward to. A lack of outward productivity. These all threaten to detach us from what we may presume to be purposeful.

However, purpose is not an objective fact but a subjective perception. Arts and crafts can redeliver a reason to move forwards in a life that has lost its previous trajectory. Each project you embark on provides something to engage with other than the trials of your body. There is a point in opening your eyes to a new day. Something achievable lies in wait for you and you alone – for nobody else will create it in exactly the way that you do.

'Get busy with life's purpose, toss aside empty hopes, get active in your own rescue,' wrote Marcus Aurelius almost two millennia ago. Spiritual doctrines teach that *being* is as important as *doing* – that our self-worth needn't be bound up in our external actions – and there is much truth in this. We lose no intrinsic value by being unproductive or by simply being. However, our identity likes to perceive a purposeful channel for itself. So much so that how well we thrive amid suffering is dictated, at least in part, by finding personal meaning.

> *Arts and crafts can redeliver a reason to move forwards in a life that has lost its previous trajectory.*

Viktor E Frankl, a survivor of Auschwitz, discovered that those most likely to survive such a horror were the people who had a future-bound personal incentive to survive – a loved one to be reunited with, a task to fulfil, a reason to keep moving onwards through the unimaginable. He concluded that survival doesn't so much hinge on *how* to make it through, but on the meaning one puts on *why* it is important to do so. This professor of neurology and psychiatry went on to detail three routes for finding personal meaning in life. Luckily for us, all three can be accessed through arts and crafts.

The first is by performing a purposeful deed or involving oneself in work. The power that creating a work of art can have on one's sense of purpose is exemplified by Shantel. After over a decade of ill health, she explains how artwork has filled the gap left by her pre-illness meaningful activities: 'I mourn the old me, but one thing that gets me through and gives me a purpose in life is my art. When I complete a piece I feel a huge sense of achievement, much like I did when I'd completed a run or a workout.' Corrine, a bedbound artist, found similar. Until she began producing self-portraits, her identity resided in being an ill person who didn't connect with any personal purpose. Now she considers herself an artist with a sense of accomplishment.

Frankl's second route to finding meaning is through love. By finding a hobby that you love to engage in, making items that you enjoy having around you, creating gifts for loved ones or producing items with compassion for charities and people in need, you are fulfilling your human need to share and feel love. When love comes into the equation, surviving becomes thriving.

But the most important route, according to Frankl, is to create triumph from tragedy. He saw that, while situations are often not under an individual's control, their attitude around the situation is theirs to choose. If constructive meaning or outcomes from the suffering can be found, then a degree of fortitude to cope with further trials is nurtured. While the inspiration for Frankl's work came from time spent in concentration camps, he is clear that what he learned is relevant to any form of suffering, without judgement of its severity.

So, how can your physical, mental and emotional pains, frustrations and limitations become your triumph? Developing a beneficial attitude in the face of relentless internal symptoms and imbalances is not easy, especially when those very symptoms may seek to alter our personality. However, there will be something you have gained, developed, learned or experienced of a positive nature due to your enforced circumstance – if only the discovery of a new creative hobby. Your use of colours, textures, words and imagery in your creations is where you can begin to practise triumphing over tragedy. Play with constructive and uplifting concepts at first. Tease them out of yourself and see how they feel to you without committing to them. Absorb them as you depict them, allowing them to influence your emotions and lift you, if only temporarily, beyond the monotony of suffering. This isn't a suggestion to ignore reality and plunge into toxic positivity but to balance the difficulties you're enduring with awareness of the (sometimes deeply) hidden gifts that accompany them.

You can also develop a triumphant sense of purpose when your condition allows you to spend time creating things that are needed by yourself or others. Make things that excite pride in how you cope with your circumstances.

Meaningful creativity

Suffering can at times feel like a punishment, at others utterly senseless, but using it creatively is one way of manifesting a constructive meaning to your situation. Perhaps arts and crafts offer a pathway of expression, lend strength to your voice, increase public awareness or become a way to share kindness? Attending as often as possible to our chosen craft, allowing it to develop significance for us, is a strong way of finding meaning within ongoing illness. Does your craft bring you joy? Comfort? Respite? These are all meaningful responses.

If you feel your motivation tank running dry, allow others who exhibit purposeful enthusiasm to infect you. Reading a small American magazine for families living in tune with nature was a turning point for me when I was almost completely bedbound and unable to parent my young daughter as I had hoped. I had imagined myself as a barefoot mama, carrying my baby through forests and fields, introducing her to the natural world. As it turned out, I couldn't even be her primary carer at home. It was heart-breaking.

I needed a way to reclaim my path through motherhood and assert my intentions, even if I couldn't enact them. It took a few years after my daughter's birth before I became well enough again to read, sit up in bed and type or draw, but in time, inspired by the American magazine I had discovered and with the blessing of that publication's editor, I created a UK magazine for families raising their children in a nature-based lifestyle. It featured songs, crafts, recipes, stories, puzzles and more that represented the mother I wanted to be. I encouraged my daughter to contribute illustrations and I shared alternative ways that I had nurtured our relationship. I had found an outlet for my creativity that held real meaning for me. It solidified my identity and reminded me of who I was beyond my condition. I was more than just an ill body in a bed.

One day a carer arrived, saw me in bed using my laptop and remarked, 'Oh, you're playing'. But I knew otherwise. I was at work. I had purpose. Some find their own meaning and purpose in gaming, the creation of virtual realities and all kinds of activities that may be seen as purely recreational.

If just one person appreciates what you have created or finds meaning in the process, and if that person is you, it has served a purpose.

Whether other people recognise the meaning an activity holds for you isn't necessarily relevant. If just one person appreciates what you have created or finds meaning in the process, and if that person is you, it has served a purpose.

The legacy of creativity

Chronic illness denies many the ability to conceive, or even consider parenthood, leaving people wondering what future-reaching ripples they will leave in this world. While this longing cannot be covered over by a hand-sewn quilt or lace shawl, a little consolation may be found in the thought that something you've brought into being may long outlive you. In addition, if you take up creative practices that your ancestors engaged in you are carrying on an aspect of your family lineage, creatively honouring those you have come from.

Similarly, through learning and sharing traditional skills, you can nurture the lineage of heritage crafts. Many require greater participation from new crafters to remain alive or be reborn in the world. The teachable techniques are the genes of these crafts that must be practised and passed on if they aren't to die out. By being the caretaker of traditional crafts, or preserver of memories through your art, you midwife the past into the future. You leave a legacy of a different kind.

Blogs, YouTube tutorials, Pinterest and Ravelry are perfect platforms from which to share tips, ideas and inspiration. If you're happy to part with your creations, there are groups devoted to championing chronically ill makers and raising money for charities via handmade items. A couple of these are mentioned in Appendix 2: Charity and kindness projects.

Keeping a scrapbook that documents your creative achievements, and positive responses from others when you have reached out and shared your work, serves as a reliable boost on low-morale days. I created a Facebook photo album of my creations as my personal gallery for others to peruse, and my Instagram account is solely for my creativity. Through these I feel that my creations are living their own lives and hopefully touching others.

Not so long ago I read about a funeral for a patchworker that featured her handmade quilts draped over the backs of the church pews. I now feel compelled to request something similar! What a wonderful tribute at the end of your life to host (albeit in absence – but this just reflects your experience with chronic illness, no?) a personal exhibition. A lifetime spent preparing the content for this showcase brings new depth of purpose to the urge to create.

Purpose, now and always

I find it important to ensure that I always have different-sized projects at varying stages of completion on the go so that my daily sense of purpose is maintained. Short-term projects provide a regular sense of achievement within sight. This is necessary when larger plans feel less attainable and the end-point drifts further away on an ill tide. We need to feel that there is a point in being here, now, and sometimes quick fixes and fast makes are the answer. A simultaneous long-term project is there to dip in and out of as and when we are able. It is a constant when the briefer projects come to an end and you haven't yet found a new focus. More importantly, it maintains our engagement with an orientation towards the future. It is our reason to keep looking forwards. Our deed propels us on with motivation.

Note that there is a difference between purpose associated with a constructive sense of direction and the kind of purpose that is fixed to a specific goal. The latter runs the risk of invoking stress and resulting in feelings of failure if not achieved. We needn't be accomplished artists or running successful craft businesses for there to be meaning in what we make.

I have frequently fallen into the trap of wondering what the point is when my work isn't outstanding, unique or destined to be appreciated by others. This, I now realise, is my ego fussing unnecessarily. It will continue to do so, I'm sure (this is its speciality), but I can do my best to rise above it and recognise the worth of what I'm doing. The purpose is not in excellence but in the intention and occupation. I don't practise the piano with any aim of performing, recording or composing but purely for the joy of my fingers on the keys and the combination of sounds I manage to recreate. The purpose, in this instance, is pleasure itself.

> *One meaningful act can influence someone for a lifetime.*

Creations need never be grand to find purpose. Old practice-pieces of art, completed colouring pages and textile samples are often suitable for transforming into cards, or small sections of gift-wrap. Or they may be worth saving to incorporate into more significant works later. Items given to others, no matter how small or infrequent, carry ongoing power. Your care for someone resides in that item long after it has been handed over, sharing love, compassion and support in your absence. We needn't berate ourselves for not constantly acting with purposeful focus. One meaningful act can influence someone for a lifetime. One overarching objective can carry us forwards, even when we are taking a break from active engagement.

Personal significance

So, to return to Marcus Aurelius, how will you rescue your personal purpose? Might you forge an escape route for locked away passions; make objects of practical use, items of uplifting beauty; or earn money through your creativity – either for your own needs or to donate?

As Viktor Frankl would ask, what is your *why* of survival?

Is it to partake in pleasure? Perhaps it is to share awareness of poorly represented perceptions? Is it to ease future experiences or to reframe past pain? Maybe finding ways to connect with the world is what holds significance for you. Are you a metaphorical mapmaker for those caught in the same terrain, letting them know others have been here too? Purpose is often felt when connecting with something larger than the individual self. Is your personal significance rooted simply in being part of the natural world, fostering a desire in you to promote ecology or represent nature in your creations? Do you feel purposeful when tending to the self, creating for others, or in a balance of the two? Some might find their purpose in bearing witness to the intricacies of the world, offering attention and compassion to their own experiences or those of others.

What do you want to lend even the smallest creative ability to, in order to live with awakened personal significance? Perhaps the meaning of life is to answer this question when the odds seem stacked against us. We each get to decide what gives our life purpose.

Suggested therapeutic activity
A life well lived

What would you like to be said of you after you've gone? Don't be humble. Explore this thought to identify what you would like the purpose of your life to encompass. Rather than specific life events, what values are important to you? Either in your mind or with pen and paper, brainstorm creative ways you could bring these attributes into being. How could your creations express your values on your behalf? Think creatively about how to achieve a version of your original desires that may have been scuppered by illness.

Creating purpose at a glance

- Those who feel a sense of purpose to their life find it easier to thrive in adverse circumstances.
- Purpose is personal and transient – it is up to you to decide what gives this stage of your life, or your day, purpose.
- Translating suffering into art can make a difficult experience feel more purposeful.
- Purpose can range from aiming to finish a row of stitches to improving the lives of others through your creations.
- When your health denies you the usual purposeful actions, arts and crafts can become an effective alternative. Choose pathways you love to engage with, that hold significance for you and are within your means.

Chapter 8
Making a difference

Being largely incapacitated by illness can leave one (understandably, but misguidedly) feeling a burden on others. The only difference we feel we make to other people's lives is a draining one. When intentions are stymied by ongoing ill health, there is an urge to prove that we still have a use, that our value doesn't just reside in how well we cope with being unwell: that we have something to offer. Not merely passive riders in our bodies, we need to know that our existence has a constructive impact on the world around us.

Good fiction writers ensure their protagonists don't have the plot simply happen to them but that they have agency over the course of the story's events. We are the protagonist of our own life story, and we are also co-author. We have a say in how our character develops. Our chosen creative path needn't only benefit ourselves. Through small actions with strong impact, it provides us with a chance to offer something back to society.

We have strengths, compassion and resilience that people who haven't lived with debilitating symptoms or difficult circumstances may not have developed to the same degree. We learn to find joy where others take life for granted and we fight battles that might never have entered their minds. These insights make powerful subject matter.

The unique expertise owned by the housebound became especially apparent during the COVID-19 pandemic lockdowns. While the rest of society was confused and traumatised by the new enforced circumstances, and the frightening surge of long COVID cases, we of the chronically ill and disabled communities came into our own. The rest of the world had ventured into the edges of our realm and were desperate for our coping mechanisms and altered living techniques. Our necessitated creative approach to everyday solutions became valued.

Beyond the rarity (we hope) of a global pandemic, we have much to offer. Our under-represented experiences need to be heard, to educate the wider public and healthcare professionals. Our learned compassion for suffering can be extended in solidarity to those feeling alone in their pain. We can make a positive difference to the world we live in, and our hobbies can help us do this.

Connecting, educating and integrating

A pivotal point in my own life, before my condition was more widely known, was when I read a book featuring other people's accounts of how ME affected them. The lightness that washed through me, the sensation of not being a lone sufferer, of knowing that experiences I'd misunderstood as personality faults were recognised symptoms, and the strength I felt in finally realising there was a tribe I belonged to, can't be overestimated. It had a knock-on effect throughout my personality and health management, and it made me realise the importance of spreading awareness.

Expressive arts and crafts are especially effective at raising awareness around difficult subjects as they carry less risk of coming across as a lecture, complaint or attack. They open a window onto visceral experiences that can touch others in ways that explanations don't always manage to. In this respect, social psychologist Dr Sara Konrath believes art to be a perfect Trojan horse, smuggling seeds of empathy into unsuspecting minds that just came along for the view. With our diversely collective experience, what a herd of Trojan horses we could let loose on the world!

The neurodivergent illustrator Andy J Pizza firmly believes in the difference we can make to other people through our artistic responses to life, and the importance of having faith in this. On his *Creative Pep Talk* podcast, he advises that when you hit that moment in an expressive project where you doubt the validity of what you are doing, remind yourself that representing your experience is not a luxury but a necessity – if not for yourself, then for someone who may one day encounter your work when in need of solidarity or guidance.

When I can transmute my struggles into art I don't just feel I've exorcised part of the pain; I hope that my representation of the experience can spread awareness for the benefit of others as well. Regardless of the quality of the finished piece, I upload it to social media for its message to travel. I recently did this with a collaged and charcoal piece called *Dancing on the Inside*. My charcoal depiction of a person lying down, with a dancing figure rising from their prone form, wasn't as accurate as I'd have liked. I felt nervous about sharing the piece but wanted to reach out with its sentiment. I was amazed at how many appreciated it, some saying how powerful the message was, others how strongly they identified with it. That piece of artwork won't win any awards or reduce any of the symptoms behind its inspiration, but if it consoles others traversing their own illness or raises compassion levels in those around them, then, in its own small way, my imperfect little picture has made a difference.

Through our creative representations, we have the opportunity to draw people's attention to uncommon diseases or poorly understood conditions. Our experience and knowledge seep into the wider community, potentially benefiting medical, social and personal responses to poorly researched or unusual illnesses. This also serves the purpose of better integrating disabled and chronically ill people in general into society's awareness. Meanwhile, chronically ill people themselves are presented with a mirror in which they can recognise their own experiences, feel less alone and know that they are represented.

Some years ago, an initiative called Number Squares appealed for people with

ME to produce a square in whatever medium they chose that displayed the number of years they had lived with the condition. Photographs of these – some drawn, some painted, some sewn (including my appliquéd 33) – were combined in a montage that was shared on social media to highlight the years lost to this illness. I have also contributed patchwork squares to a community-created quilt that was auctioned off to raise funds for biomedical research into ME.

Involvement in a cause needn't cease when our presence in the outside world diminishes.

Raising awareness of diverse health conditions is clearly a valid cause. The irony is that those of us with the most to share on the subject often have the least energy to make ourselves heard in traditional ways. But involvement in a cause needn't cease when health falters and our presence in the outside world diminishes. In fact, for some this is when it begins. The artist Elizabeth Jameson, who we met in Chapter 3 (page 26), had been a public-interest lawyer before developing MS. Her diagnosis didn't dent her desire to make an impact on society but it did change the way she had to do it. Now, she uses art instead of law. As her condition has worsened, she employs assistance to manifest her artistic visions in an effort to continue broadening society's narrative around illness and what it can mean to live within an ill body.

For others, further patience is required while being forced to wait for their body, or the medical system, to offer enough respite to be able to make their own difference. Jordan Plotnar founded the Resonance Project after surgery improved his quality of life with EDS enough to film a short documentary. Such an endeavour could seem intimidating to those of us unable to consider a project of this ambition, but there is room in creative activism for all levels of contribution. Jordan composed a piece of orchestral and choral music to accompany the film with the idea that anyone living anywhere with chronic illness or disability could take part by downloading the score, recording their contribution and submitting their video to him. His aim was to digitally combine these contributions and for this virtual ensemble to collaborate with his film in raising better public and clinical awareness of multiple conditions as well as hopefully provoking further medical research.

Craftivism

My textile contributions to ME awareness projects were acts of craftivism – a gentle form of activism that invites small, crafted contributions to add to collective campaigns. Finding something larger than ourselves to become involved with is a powerful affirmation of our inclusion in society. Further to this, lending our voice to communities or causes other than those that directly affect ourselves moves us out of a space where our life is dominated by our own struggles and closer to a feeling of relevance and usefulness in the wider world.

Lauren O'Farrell (also known by the fabulous moniker Deadly Knitshade) is an author, artist and pioneer of the form of craftivism known as graffiti knitting. Through her strategically placed offerings, she spreads positive messages and yarn-induced smiles. It was when she was ill with Hodgkin's lymphoma and couldn't read or write due to severe brain fog that she took up the craft she would come to use as a voice of activism.

Online organisations like the Craftivist Collective regularly select social and ecological campaigns to focus their efforts on and appeal for small hand-crafted pieces that deliver specific messages. These are then sent to MPs or CEOs or distributed randomly for members of the public to find. Kits are sold for those who require a little help in getting started on their own at home, so there is no need to attend gatherings or classes.

Internet searches around crafts and causes that are close to your heart will often reveal projects to lend your passion to. It was a Facebook post that encouraged me to contribute a simple embroidery to a patchwork banner aiming to foster a welcoming attitude towards refugees; and a Facebook group that organised a collective textile contribution to that year's Woollen

Woods display, in which we highlighted how to preserve our countryside's bee and insect population.

The generosity of devoting time and quiet patience to a carefully considered message is perhaps what makes craftivism effective where protests or demonstrations may fail to reach their target audience. These handmade items, given away with kindness and hope, touch people gently but thought-provokingly. It turns out that not being able to march with activists may not be preventing us from making a difference after all.

The definition of craftivism is that your creation addresses the root of a problem and how to stop it from happening, as opposed to donating to those already affected. But that is not to diminish the importance of the latter. It is simply another path of action. For me, the two go hand in hand.

The usefulness of creativity

While it is preferable that problems are remedied at source, gifting items directly to those in emotional or physical need can feel more immediately helpful. When Knit for Peace conducted a study on the effects of knitting items specifically to donate to charities, they learned that 65% of the participants who both knitted and were in poor health felt more useful by knitting for others. When we feel powerless over our own circumstances, the ability to facilitate comfort for others (out of choice, as and when able, rather than in response to stressful demands) is powerful emotional medicine. You have shared solace with others. The world is one act of generosity better for having you in it.

The ability to facilitate comfort for others (out of choice, as and when able, rather than in response to stressful demands) is powerful emotional medicine.

When Ellie was receiving chemotherapy for breast cancer, half a dozen or so friends in her online illness community conspired to knit a comfort blanket that she could wrap around herself during her chemo sessions. Years on, and having been given the all-clear, she still uses her blanket daily to comfort her through ongoing autoimmune symptoms. In turn, Ellie founded an online group knitting squares that she sewed into blankets for the homeless. Ellie has warmed numerous people with her blankets and hats but the effect it has had on her, the giver, is apparent when she speaks about knitting. 'I'm not especially proficient, and I'm not gifted with a talent for design, but I make useful, important things. Hats, mittens, jumpers, blankets, socks, shawls. There is something very powerful in that.'

Anna Wood discovered that, despite being predominantly housebound, her eye for nature photography needn't go to waste. By welcoming birds into her garden, she gathered a collection of images worthy of forming a book. *25 Birds – One Year, One Garden* has not only brought birdlife into the laps of many others living with chronic illness but, with the profits all being donated to charity, has already raised hundreds of pounds to fund biomedical research into ME – the illness Anna suffers from.

Feeling able to give as well as receive, to make as well as take, is important. Those around you already know that you are far more than your body's needs, that you are wholly meaningful in your own right. However, sometimes we need to remind ourselves. What better way than by knowing that your creative act will be held and used by another human in need of your compassion?

Appendix 2 on 'Charity and kindness projects', in Part 6, lists a selection of charities, groups and organisations appealing for handmade donations. Some also welcome materials that others can use, either in their gifted creations or by community welfare projects. This is another way for us to contribute, even when too unwell to make something ourselves.

Doing something in service to others, no matter how small, affirms to ourselves that we have something valuable to contribute. Through our creative generosity we get to provide something of use (practically or emotionally) to someone in need, and who isn't in need in one way or another?

The difference kindness makes

Making a difference doesn't require staying in a constant space of productivity. I dip in and out of the energy and motivation to make items for social campaigns, and trust that what I do, when I do it, is enough. We must balance sharing kindness in the outer world with being kind to ourselves: making the difference between surviving and thriving in our own sphere of existence, as well as seeking to help others. Not that giving to others is an entirely altruistic act. Research has demonstrated that both performing, and recollecting, acts of kindness can have a beneficial effect on the giver, with the potential to improve immune function, lower stress hormones, instigate feelings of meaningful happiness and release oxytocin (the hormone that helps us feel bonded with others as well as having cardiovascular benefits).

Ruth cares about humanitarian causes and making the world a fairer place. Bedbound with severe ME and limited in how she can play a part in bettering the world, she still has ways. When able, she creates digital art from her sickbed. Whether painting a memorial for a lost member of her illness community, promoting an animal charity, or offering a free-to-share image raising political awareness, she uses her art compassionately. I barely knew Ruth when she gifted me, via social media, a portrait of my cat who had just died. The consideration she had put into using her limited energy to recreate my much-missed companion deeply touched me. It made the world feel a warmer place, and the personal enjoyment she experienced was an added layer to the value of the act.

There is no hierarchy of importance about who you support, what you create or how long its lifespan will be. It could be a card for a loved one; a heart for a lonely friend to hold; home-baked thank-you biscuits for a health- or care-worker; a story of hope and solidarity for someone who is struggling. A photo book of uplifting images to be left in a waiting room, welcome gifts for refugees or items for post-operative patients all reach out into the world on your behalf, sometimes further than originally imagined. Who knows what future kindnesses and strength they will foster as well as their immediate comfort?

When I learned about Bobby Buddies (teddies to be handed out by the police to traumatised children), I had enthusiastic visions of knitting a whole constabulary of dozens for our local police force. The time they took me to complete, combined with the effect on my hands meant that I ended up making just two. In time I am sure I will make more. In the meantime, two children have been shown a kindness. I was told by a friend that she couldn't put that amount of work into something that might end up being thrown in a muddy puddle. I pointed out that if a distressed child gained any relief by throwing the teddy across the road or picking it to pieces, then my efforts had served their purpose. My expectation of how a gift of kindness will be used is irrelevant in the face of the recipient's needs.

For a while I made kindness bookmarks. These were simple strips of card that I decorated in colourful pens with patterns and suggestions of random acts of kindness. Sentiments such as, 'You are more loved than you know' with 'Share the love' on the reverse, and 'Anyone who takes time to be kind is beautiful', were placed in books being returned to the library, dropped off at charity shops or left at book swaps. It excited me to think that somebody would discover a bookmark and feel they had found a little treasure to keep. That alone might make them smile, which is what making a difference is all about. If the hand-lettered suggestions and phrases inspired them to commit their own acts of kindness (for themselves or others), then a train of events had been set in motion by my tiny creation.

More recently, I contributed to a collective aiming to brighten the streets of war-torn Kyiv by making some paper-collaged bunting pennants to be pasted on their walls. I had been in a severe health crash and unable to craft at all for a couple of months but now found myself able to sit up in bed and fiddle with scraps of paper. It was deeply rewarding to sift through old magazines and calendars for nature pictures and patterns, cutting and tearing and rearranging without any pressure for a perfect finish – simply using my hands to deliver aesthetic support to people I would never know.

We get to make a difference by reminding another human being that they are appreciated, considered, recognised and cared about. The value of this must never be under-estimated. An American study showed that when patients discharged from hospital following suicidal ideation received caring letters that expressed a desire to stay in contact, they were less likely to attempt suicide again. A handmade card or decorated letter could mean more to the recipient than you will ever know. Of course, your gift needn't be something you physically hand over but may be your time and encouragement, sharing skills and facilitating another's creative response to life.

> *When I am so unwell that I wonder how to carry on, I remember how I have made a difference in the past and I plan future ways to share creative kindness.*

Making a difference doesn't always take place in the way we expect it to. Our involvement is what matters. Once we set the kindness free, it can travel anywhere, sometimes back to ourselves. Focusing on helping another can lessen isolated immersion in our own struggles, making a single crafted kindness a double-strength act.

When I am so unwell that I wonder how to carry on, I remember how I have made a difference to people in the past through creating items for charities and individuals. I plan future ways to share creative kindness, and I know that if I can lift the spirits of just one person, then I have achieved something above and beyond surviving my illness.

Suggested creative exercise
The power of you

Make a list of those whose lives you would like to make a difference to. These could be individuals who are close to you, care workers you encounter, groups of people, future generations, animals…

Now list the ways in which you could realistically be of positive impact. These might include sending a voice note of you singing a song to remind them you care, writing a letter of appreciation, or a card of encouragement; spreading awareness, fundraising, creating useful items; or any other creative offering of support that you can come up with. Appendix 2's list of charities and causes seeking handcrafted contributions may help you with this.

Choose one of the recipients on your list, select an action you can take, and get started when you next feel able.

Making a difference at a glance

- Feeling that we are having a positive impact on the world is important when so reduced in capacity. We need to feel that we are giving as well as taking support.
- We have more to offer than we sometimes give ourselves credit for.
- Creations focusing on our experience help others going through similar and feeling alone.
- We can raise awareness around health conditions, communicating information and opportunities for empathy through our arts and crafts.
- Crafts can be employed in service to a number of important causes, from ecology to kindness to social activism, locally and abroad.
- Even occasional acts of crafty kindness make an impact on the giver and the receiver. The effect of your gift to others doesn't end when you hand it over.
- Turn to the list of Charity and kindness projects in Appendix 2 (page 315) for ideas of how to make a difference through your creativity.

Chapter 9
Creative connections

Illness is a land of its own, where certain rules and etiquette apply. Our behaviour evolves to suit the unique terrain, with its concealed sinkholes and hidden dangers. And, while the language may sound like that of neighbouring lands, some words resembling those used in the healthy world hold painfully different meanings, leaving us often struggling to be understood or to connect with those who haven't resided here.

When chronically ill, we frequently require quietude and stillness to replenish easily depleted energy reserves, and yet humanity is a tribal species, living in closely connected groups for physical and emotional wellbeing. The isolation that can accompany long-term ill health, then, is often a central source of conflict.

In fact, as anyone who has lived in long-term isolating circumstances will know, the pain of loneliness can burrow far deeper than physical discomforts, chewing away and distorting the shape of our self-perception. When healthy people's lives are consumed with work, family and their own leisure commitments, it is all too easy for us to feel forgotten, stranded on our quiet Isle of Illness, out of sight and, perhaps, out of mind. Even when we are remembered by the mainlanders, we may doubt that we will ever fully belong with the healthy tribe. Where are the people like us, who we can be ourselves with, without searching for ways to convey our extreme experiences, or something other than health to talk about because we don't want to alienate ourselves further? They are on their own islands.

We may once have been sociable extroverts but now here we are, often alone, frequently lonely and without workaday conversational topics to fall back on. Our lives revolve around a subject that healthy people rarely want to dwell on. To be honest, it's one we'd rather not focus on so much, either. Support groups are valuable but have their limitations. We long for relationships that connect through hobbies and enjoyment as much as enforced experience. Life and friendship should surely encompass more than just illness, shouldn't they?

I have painted this gloomy picture because it has been my experience in the past and one that I'm aware many others are living. However, we can add highlights to the scene. As we explored in the previous two chapters, even when unable to move our bodies closer to other people, our creative output reaches out on our behalf. Knit for Peace have concluded that those who knit items for others experience an increased sense of inclusion in society and a reduction in loneliness and isolation. A little creativity can travel a long way to join us with others. Role models, like-minded groups, and new friends we can share our chosen interests with are all within creative reach. We just need the shared language of creativity.

Online connections

The time of least creative inspiration for me was when housebound before the internet and social media became widespread. I feared that fresh motivation would be beyond me for as long as I was confined to my home. However, in time, my creativity began flowing richly again through a Facebook group for chronically ill people with creative urges. In my own time, at my own pace, with or without active involvement, I could absorb the stimuli of a plethora of creations, thought processes and influences. Here at my fingertips was an outpouring of creative minds that I could filter through my own individuality. My motivation was fed.

Technology has been wonderful in bringing us closer to each other without requiring our bodies to leave our homes. Book groups, craft and chronic illness groups, stitch-alongs, art workshops and choirs are all available to attend from your home, in your pyjamas if necessary.

Handicrafts have seen a renaissance that is in full swing, and the accessibility of creative hobbies for those of us living a largely disabled life means that communities combining these two features are a natural result. With internet searches revealing virtual assemblies all around the world, you will inevitably find a community that suits you.

I have felt a connection with others even when too weak to speak or smile by joining an online event with my microphone and camera turned off so I can lie with my eyes shut, listening to the conversation and hearing myself welcomed by participants who know how ill I am and appreciate my presence, even if I contribute no more than a name on a screen.

Just following other people in the illness community on social media reminds us that we are not alone: that we are connected even in our separation. And, of course, following completely healthy artists and crafters online brings their work and their communications to us when unable to attend exhibitions, classes or workshops. All kinds of communities become accessible when reached via cyberspace.

Even those who shy away from the over-stimulation that social media can exert might find a gentle, cushioned corner of the internet in creativity groups, especially those aimed at members who are also chronically ill. There is an air of compassion, encouragement, understanding and escapism in these virtual spaces. Appendix 3: Online Resources, in Part 6, will lead you to some that I have found supportive and creatively inspiring.

It's true that communicating via technology is no replacement for the physical presence of another person, especially for affectionate touch, but I have found it to come a very close second and it brings its own advantages (being able to switch off the screen the moment interaction becomes too much, being one!). Some have postulated that singing can help make up for lack of bodily contact, in which case an online choir is ideal for isolated people craving a more physical connection. It is also noted that both stroke and dementia patients who have lost their power of fluent speech can often remember song lyrics and sing with ease, making this activity a possibility for those who struggle with concentrating on conversations.

Singing can help make up for lack of physical contact.

Whenever the body is able, the arts and creativity are valuable communication and connection pathways for those with any illness that causes isolation, brain fog or speech difficulties. While I and my ill friends rarely synchronise windows of energy for telephone calls, we do leave each other short voice messages, listening and responding in our own time. My voice-messaging friends and I have little or no work life, and few social or leisure events to discuss, but we connect over our creative strategies for living life as fully as we can. And when even this falters? When coherent speech or constructive thought becomes too much? Like singing, the ability to create art has also been seen to remain in people with dementia or neurological conditions long after speech and language faculties have diminished. We send each other photos of finished art pieces, and of the creations woven by nature outside our windows or brought to our bedsides. We photograph works in progress, newly acquired materials, patterns discovered, and examples of inspiring (or hilarious) pieces found online. No (or few) words are needed to communicate that we are still here, we are more than our illness and we are thinking of each other. As my online friend Lior once wrote to me: 'Having seen something you've created is part of knowing you better. Helpful when neither of us has much capacity to talk.'

We are aware that our symptoms are shouting but we quietly affirm hope, humour and solidarity, sharing personalities that connect with each other in more than the arbitrariness of a shared diagnosis.

The power of community

Dwelling in my own head so much of the time, over-familiar with my own company and thought patterns, I feel exhilarated when I have shared a connection with someone else. At times it is like taking a temporary holiday from myself and seeing new views. On other occasions, I get to perceive myself anew, through another's eyes, through shared experience and greater understanding.

A good community binds together to solve problems, offer guidance and share ideas, motivation, distraction and friendship. They refresh faded laughter and strengths. Its members hold hands, forming a circle that is more powerful than the sum of its parts but richer for each individual component. Making tangible items for or with a community augments this affirmation of belonging and connecting. The added benefit of an artistic community is that it celebrates an aspect of ourselves that illness hasn't entirely stomped over (for, even if too unwell to create our own art, we can still appreciate that of others) or perhaps has even uncovered. However, it needn't be a specifically artistic community to nurture that aspect of ourselves. Jo loves to draw the objects around her but, being bedbound, she was finding that 'sadness, loneliness and loss start to seep out when I try drawing my own environment.' So, Jo reached out to an online illness support group. She requested photos from other people's bedsides and windows that she could use as a basis for her drawings, when well enough, and her sense of shared experience. Photographs of objects, animals, plants and views filled the screen as members of her community embraced this way of helping a fellow sufferer.

Whatever community you identify with, what matters is a sense of belonging. Clinging to a community that no longer serves or welcomes us is counterproductive. Instead, we can congregate with those who understand and affirm the life we are living.

I told Anna, a friend I met through the online ME/CFS community, that I use a reward chart to motivate myself to stay within my safe limits when tempted to let enthusiasm spur me into too much activity. In the past, I'd felt alone in having to curtail fun simply to lie down and do nothing. I resented it. However, texting her one lunchtime to say that my happy news for the day was feeling able to schedule a writing session for that afternoon, she typed back, 'Yay for writing! I want to hear that you have a gold star later for sticking to your time.' Instead of begrudging that I had to limit how long I would write for, my awareness was redirected towards what I *could* do. My technique for looking after my health had been embraced by someone who understood the need for it and welcomed the fun challenge. Since then, we have awarded each other stars via texts in support of self-restraint in the interest of longer-term quality of health.

Rather than feeling like you alone must prioritise healthcare to such an extent, having someone else out there who reflects your situation reminds you that you're not an outcast, just a member of a different societal club. We are not alone. There is strength in that. While a lone stick of chalk can be readily broken, hold many together in a group and they are harder to snap. And it turns out that the chronically ill community contains many more of us than I had imagined during my younger years of living with ill health.

Those living with debilitating conditions usually have a desire to find others who are going through similar, tending to be communicative about what they're experiencing and receptive to others reaching out. Similarly, members of the online creative communities that I have settled in are eager to share, help and encourage. These parallels in the chronic illness and creative communities are perfect foundations for potentially strong relationships.

Our crafts become our social glue, mediator and communal therapy.

By joining together with both a shared appreciation of crafts and mutual understanding of life with chronic illness, we discover friendship and support in people we might not otherwise have approached. Strands of previously unrecognised connections are given the opportunity to bond. Sharing difficult experiences, virtually or in person, is made less intense or overwhelming when we have the diversion of our chosen crafts to turn to. We can slide from concern and care to light-hearted craft-talk as the moment dictates. We can contribute what we are capable of without dreading awkward silences; listen to each other without pressure to instantly respond. Our crafts become our social glue, mediator and communal therapy.

S-J lives in a dimly lit room with severe ME. Her condition has stripped her of virtually all of her creative abilities, so she seeks new ways to involve herself in creative entertainment. One option that works for her is to start a story game on social media where she offers an opening word or sentence and others pitch in to take the story forward, sentence by sentence. S-J joins in as she's able, feeling a part of this community story that she has instigated. She also interacts with Artificial Intelligence (AI) to produce text, pictures and colouring pages that she couldn't otherwise realise, again reaching out to her online community for suggestions of what they'd like to see. AI is a controversial topic, especially in the art world, but S-J is proof of its value in the disabled community and, used appropriately, its ability to nurture human connections. 'Having an arty hobby again, especially making pictures, poems and stories for others, has really helped my mental health,' she says.

Low self-esteem is especially easy to slip into when isolated from a supportive community. This is exacerbated when we struggle physically in areas of life that most others are able to take for granted. We hover on the edge of society, often only being seen when our body allows us to exceed what we generally find sustainable. We then run the risk of finding ourselves either overly praised for bravery or accused of faking our illness.

Either way, we're left feeling a disconnect between perceptions (held by ourselves as well as others) and the reality of the situation. When dissonance like this becomes so ingrained as to become part of our identity, we can naturally transfer it to all pursuits we take up. We can begin to imagine that we aren't creative at all, rather than merely in need of input, especially when deprived of an immersive community to share ideas and feedback with.

It is all too easy to feel like an imposter in the world of arts and crafts unless we hear from others who have experienced similar struggles, mistakes and doubts, and risen to the challenge. Other people's enthusiasm and motivation are infectious, especially when they are encountering similar difficulties and obstacles.

Hidden collaborations

If you find accessing online communities and events beyond your current abilities, don't despair. A sense of shared outcome can still be fostered by being mindful of the origins of the creative materials you use and who else may be engaged in the same project elsewhere. Even propped up alone in bed, colouring in a pre-drawn picture, working from a craft kit or piecing together a jigsaw puzzle is a collaborative act with its originator. Somebody drew the design for you to complete. Somewhere out there are other people embellishing it with their own visions of colour and technique. You are united in your activity. While this kind of connection is no replacement for company and expressed solidarity, it is a way to feel a connection with other creative people when severe ill health isolates you from more tangible communities.

Sharing our stories

A community needn't be held together by location or coordinated communication. It can span time and space through shared stories (literal or metaphorically contained in handcrafted creations), offered out to be received by others elsewhere.

Translating tangled ineffable emotions into a captured moment to be recognised by somebody else, anywhere at any time, isn't curative but it holds potential to be an emotionally healing act. Art that represents the seemingly inexpressible throws out a lifeline to and from the depths. We feel a weight lift as we release ourselves from carrying the fullness of our story internally and solitarily. The sucking whirlpool of aloneness loosens its grip a little. By reaching out to communicate our experience through fact, fiction, image or any combination of these, we reduce the sense of drowning in the immersion of our lived experience. We are waving to others in the same waters or to those at the shoreline.

When prosaic words are overwhelmed by the swollen waves of illness, creative expression enables our story to be seen. Paula Knight is an illustrator who has turned her focus towards writing since becoming bedbound with ME and PoTS. 'People with my conditions are often treated as unreliable narrators of their bodily experience,' she says, in an interview she gave for the Big Draw entitled 'Take a Line for A Lie Down'. 'So drawing and writing can become evidence and self-advocacy.'

Even when I haven't publicly exposed work of this kind, I've felt a relief in regurgitating a personally oppressive experience to be examined more objectively and then set aside from further ruminations. Turning it into something tangible, it is available at any point in the future when the need to feel witnessed or offer solidarity is strong. With it stored in preparation for sharing, I can stop circling around the experience so intently, wondering if and how, should the opportunity arise, I can do justice to the telling of my story. I can let my mind rest elsewhere. I can allow myself to move beyond negative experience.

If you do feel able to share your work, those who encounter and identify with it will feel relief at discovering they are not uniquely afflicted. You may even touch a part of someone else's experience that they were only subliminally aware of. In instigating such awareness, you are opening a pathway for compassion, relief and understanding. It becomes implicitly suggested that if you can navigate this, then perhaps they can too. At the very least, solidarity can offer some consolation.

Through a collective outpouring of stories, we demonstrate that we are not an isolated voice and thus have greater influence on communities we intersect with. Dr Annie Brewster recognises the power of art to express one's story.

As a patient with MS, she is also acutely aware of the importance of feeling properly heard by healthcare professionals. Her initiative, the Health Story Collaborative, provides an outlet for people to share their experiences in written, audio or artistic form. She firmly believes in the therapeutic effect for both the storyteller and the reader or listener and uses these personal narratives to help educate others.

Focusing on specific narratives, as opposed to generalisations or dry facts and figures, brings different existences more viscerally to life where they are remembered more easily. Personal stories hold power. Shared and heard well, they are fertiliser for growth.

Even people with a matching diagnosis will experience and respond to their condition differently. Offering up and paying attention to each other's take on the story helps everyone to expand their perspective, compassion and coping strategies. Clare Patey of the Empathy Museum makes the case for the transformative power of storytelling by reminding us that we learn to see the world differently through other people's stories. Our viewpoint widens.

Don't be put off by the use of the word 'story' here. Our stories can be conveyed in all manner of media. Through a mutual online friend, I was introduced to Vi, an artist living with chronic illness who shares her personal experiences and compassionate messages via simple captioned drawings. An opportunity for collaborative art was facilitated by social media when Vi asked permission to combine a sentence of mine with a drawing that it had inspired her to produce. Her characters are purposefully anatomically incorrect, conveying both a freedom from conventionality and a naïve style that focuses the attention on the message rather than the artwork itself. My throwaway comment and her urge to illustrate it combined to create a sense of togetherness and a path towards greater understanding of our individual experiences.

> *I decided that artistic ability wasn't to be an issue. The results surprised me.*

Around this time, during a health phase that put my sewing machine, knitting needles, paints and long-form writing beyond reach, Vi's online creative contributions inspired me to give basic strip cartoons a go. I had been feeling isolated in the severity of my health struggles and in need of expression, so decided that artistic ability wasn't to be an issue. I would let myself combine simple stick characters and short phrases to express myself, without aspiring to anything greater. The results surprised me. My drawings were sufficient and when sharing them online I felt seen, the direct and unassuming images seeming to connect with others without need for so much cognitive work on either my part or theirs.

When representing our most deeply felt nature we are more likely to find others whose interior world resonates with our own. Through the outreach of stories, strangers become allies. Opening the curtains on not just our illness but on occluded aspects of our personality affirms our multi-faceted character. We are more than just our illness; sharing the layered stories of ourselves can help others to recognise that.

Maintaining contact

Staving off loneliness requires more than brief connections or simply sending our creativity out into the world. We want to nurture two-way relationships that deepen over time.

Regularly attending craft sessions, as well as volunteering to help run groups or workshops for any age or ability, is one way to establish yourself within a community. If you are well enough and inclined in this way, investigate what's on, or could be hosted, at local libraries, community centres, craft shops, churches or private homes.

But how do we maintain connections and strengthen the delicate shoots of friendship when unable to consistently join in?

One way of remaining present with in-person groups without always attending is to initiate a text conversation or social media group in which each session's main topics are summarised and progress made in-between meet-ups is shared via discussions and photographs. This way you stay in the loop and demonstrate your enthusiasm as a member, even when unable to attend in person.

A digital newsletter or paper-zine embracing a group identity, that members can submit to if they wish, might add an enjoyable dimension that encourages participation from those who can only attend gatherings sporadically. Through a collaboration that doesn't require in-person appearance, their presence is integrated and appreciated. It may be that you could put this together from your home, thus finding an inclusive creative role even in your physical absence.

Make online creativity groups regular haunts of yours so that names and personalities become familiar and yours is as recognised as anyone else's. It doesn't matter if you have no creative evidence of your own to submit. Peruse other people's contributions, enjoy their offerings and leave supportive feedback. By simply contributing hearts of appreciation, you are participating. By gaining inspiration, enjoyment or education you are a valid member. In time you may feel able to share a bit about yourself, upload past creations or the inklings of future ideas. Remind yourself through continued, if intermittent, interaction how the group benefits from your involvement as much as you do from being a member.

Maintaining contact with other arty-crafty types can take the form of art exchanges where you create postcard-sized art to post to each other. Another version of this is to become journal buddies. In this scenario, everyone involved has a journal that all contribute to – writing, drawing, doodling or collaging in it when it is their turn to receive it in the post – before sending it on to the next person. This can be carried out with a single journal that travels from participant to participant or back and forth between two people, but

Chapter 9

by having as many journals as there are participants anyone can contribute at any time, even if another member is too unwell to pass their journal on for a while. Swap as regularly with each other as suits all parties so that the books are full of alternating creative offerings. You will learn creatively from each other and feel part of a shared endeavour. You may even get to see how others have illustrated your words or added text inspired by your pictures, discovering how your interactions with each other unearth new directions. Artistic talent isn't necessary, just interest and enthusiasm.

Not all your friends will share your involvement with creative pursuits, but most people appreciate creative offerings. During the COVID-19 pandemic I created a party in a box for family members who were self-isolating over Christmas. More recently, I parcelled up a holiday in a box for a housebound friend who loves Cornwall. In his packaged holiday I included pictures and postcards, a recipe for Cornish pasties, a list of films set in the area that he could choose from to watch online, Cornish fudge and ale, and a tiny pewter Cornish pixie. I wrote out web addresses for an online tour of a Cornish art gallery, live beach-view webcams, and a pub where he could imagine himself lodging. A short guided-imagery story described the scenery and schedule, weaving the accompanying items into the order of events. The sending and receiving of this holiday in a box was rewarding for both of us and our friendship.

I connect with healthy friends and family in a similar way to my relationships with worldwide ill friends. Sharing online or via text a photograph of a recent creation that I think will appeal, or my latest poem or short story, keeps the channels of relationship open. Without struggling to find a shared experience to chat about, an explanation of why communication is hard right now, or when I just want to connect without verbalisation of anything specific, this is my standby method of communication. Just a link to an artist or book I think they will appreciate suffices when I have nothing of my own to share.

When up to it, I make small gifts (a crocheted heart, for example, for someone I know is feeling isolated), cards or illustrated snail mail for those I can't see in person. Cookies and cake sent by post have so far arrived in one piece and are always appreciated. No matter if an assistant has carried out the majority of the work. If it's your idea, your twist on a recipe or your wishes whispered into the mixture then your creative spirit is reaching out in friendship. Even when interacting socially in more usual ways is beyond our physical capacity, our quiet creativity can reach out on our behalf, reminding friends and family that we are still here, thinking and caring about them.

On occasion, when up to the task, I have recorded myself reading poetry or book excerpts for unwell friends and they have done the same for me. How comforting it is to have the voice of a friend reading stories at your bedside. And how fulfilling to know that you are there, at least in intention and audio form, for them.

Similarly, when my daughter was very young and I was too weak to regularly read her bedtime stories, in my strong-enough moments I recorded myself reading her favourite books. At bedtime we would snuggle up together and listen to me reading while she looked at the pictures on the pages or drifted off to sleep. One night, when she couldn't sleep, I heard from another room my familiar recorded words saying 'Night night. I love you,' to which her sleepy little voice responded, 'I love you too, Mummy'. Despite my regularly having to lie with my eyes shut in a separate space from her, I had created a way to be more than just an ill member of the household and to affirm my role as her mum.

Suggested therapeutic activity
Connections

Make a list of people you would like to foster a closer connection with. This might include family members or friends you have fallen out of regular contact with, or people you have never known well but would like to forge more of a relationship with. Or perhaps you'd like to meet new people in the chronic illness community, or fellow crafters.

Brainstorm ways you could encourage a flow of contact. Consider what you could photograph, draw or make for individuals, or what other artists' and creators' work they might enjoy you sharing with them. Is there somebody on your list (or a group or social media audience) you could begin a pen-friendship, shared project or art challenge with? You needn't be working on the same item or to the same timescale to share progress reports, feelings and experiences along the way.

Now, reach out. Don't take it to heart if it doesn't work out with the first person or group you choose. Consider this an experiment. It's not crucial that it pans out how you'd hoped. In fact, it may take a while to find the people that you connect best with, and who are in a position to reciprocate (it took me years), but when you do it will be worth it.

Creative connections at a glance

- Being reminded that we belong to a community, no matter how disparate, is a valuable antidote to the loneliness and isolation that chronic illness sufferers can feel.
- Finding a creative tribe within the chronic illness community is one route for developing friendships without the focus being only on ill health.
- Sharing arts and crafts (your own or others') is a way of staying in touch with people when your own capacity for communication, or repertoire of conversational topics, is depleted.
- We are emotionally strengthened by constructive connections with others, especially when supporting each other creatively.
- Sharing our personal story can be simultaneously cathartic for ourselves and comforting and informative for others.
- The list of 'Online Resources' in Appendix 3 (see page 321) contains online groups and virtual get-togethers for the chronically ill who are creatively inclined.

Part 4:

Crafting your path

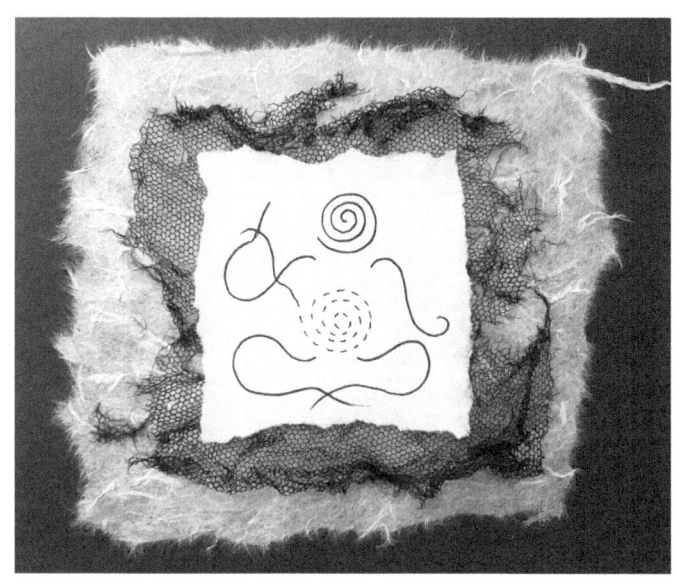

Chapter 10
Spinning gold from straw

If you have recently become ill your regular patterns of living are being broken down. When anything is dismantled it is an opportunity to not just aim for reconstruction but welcome unexplored possibilities. Your familiar daily schedule may have been pulled from under your feet, but in its wake is released the chance to turn your attention to hobbies that a busy, healthy life may not have found time for. And it's not just the way you fill your time that changes. Everything risks being disrupted, down to the very identity we had shaped for ourselves. Here, too, we can seek the positives to be mined from our situation, for when the old has been knocked down to its foundations there is space and motivation to embark on a creative re-build. What is a blockade to one way of being can become a gateway to another, when creativity is employed.

> *What is a blockade to one way of being can become a gateway to another.*

Obstructive barriers are often what improves art, forcing innovative ideas. Flash fiction, sonnets and haiku are examples of deliberately imposed restrictions on word count and format that result in powerful writing. I have found that giving myself a very specific criteria of precisely 250 words when crafting flash fiction forces me to cast out extraneous words and experiment more with my use of language. The results are more satisfying, for me, than when writing without limitation. And in the world of film making, it is legendary that George A Romero's films were so successful because his financial constraints forced him to think more creatively than directors who had money to fall back on.

Life with chronic illness is, in so many ways, restricted. It is conducted outside the inner circle of society, where all the action is, but rather than inhibiting creative output it might make it more original. Being, to some extent, an outsider has the benefit of allowing one to develop personal expression and perspectives less influenced by popular behaviour or expectations. Artifice is stripped away and space is freed up for one's deepest self to command centre stage. Mozart was known to say, "When I am ... completely myself, entirely alone ... or during the night when I cannot sleep, it is on such occasions that my ideas flow best and most abundantly."

Solitude and insomnia, reduced financial income, removal from the heart of societal functions – these familiar aspects of chronic illness are just a few of the raw materials for our creative gold.

Original vantage points

Consider the unique, honed life that your condition is forcing you to live. There is no substitute for fine health and free flung fun; I know this. However, a constructive perspective that views one's life as a work of art, forged from the imposition of illness is one way of accepting our circumstances and recognising the beauty in this unchosen colour palette. It may initiate a new understanding of oneself, of recalibrated priorities and interests, which in turn can feed back into our creations.

Illness and disability naturally provide different perspectives. We are not living as the majority do. Sitting in a wheelchair puts my line of sight at a different level from how urban environments are designed to be experienced. Being parked in my chair facing a direction I wouldn't have chosen for myself forces me to absorb what's in front of me rather than what habit would have me notice. Lying on the ground when I suddenly need to be prone, I see the world from new angles.

Moving around more slowly than others, and extended periods of being in bed, alter perceptions of time and motion. Resting in fading daylight or watching shadows move and change, without the distraction of personal activity, invites me to recognise shadows and patterns I might otherwise not observe. Having my brain amplify light and sound, translating them into physical discomfort, offers new experiences to potentially include in creative expression.

According to psychologist and art historian Tobi Zausner, for people living with the rare condition of complete colour blindness, seeing the world in monochrome can augment their tone perception. This reinforces the notion that a deficiency or difficulty in one area of life can lead to adaptive strengths. What tonal qualities in life are you more aware of since sharing your life with chronic illness? How can you use the experiences specific to your life with chronic illness to tap into original perspectives and creative visions?

Physical discomfort offers new experiences to include in creative expression.

Look at everyday objects around you, weeds in the garden, cloud patterns outside the window, and textures in detail. Investigate sensations in your body and how they migrate, cluster and change. Paying close attention is what makes a good artist. Being deprived of vast vistas needn't deprive you of artistic influences. Instead, it encourages you to look as if through a microscope at your own quadrant of life – something that nobody but you can do. When denied access to the great outdoors or big ambitions, focus your attention on what you do have and embellish the details with your own perceptions.

Transforming life's raw ingredients

Being confined by illness, unable to explore wild horizons or plan freely for the future, forces us to pay attention to the here and now. It may at times feel boring, mundane and repetitive but it is up to us to honour these feelings and then search beyond them. A dash of creative humour or a surreal slant almost always improves the moment. With or without a sense of humour, through a considered response the ordinary can become extraordinary, the raw ingredients more palatable than they at first appear. Remain open to possibility and you will find rewards in this different life to the one you were planning.

From my mid-twenties to mid-thirties I required carers to look after both me and my daughter. Some stayed with us for long enough to feel like additions to our family, others came and went with distressing frequency. It was hard to adapt to strangers in our home looking after our basic needs, especially when almost every dinner we ate for a decade was reliant on their cooking ability. We encountered carers who struggled to cook edible pasta or were mesmerised by spices and, while I had recipes and basic cooking knowledge, I was frequently too unwell to communicate these to whoever was taking care of us. We also had carers who brightened our mealtimes with traditional and original recipes from their own heritage or lifestyle. I wanted to carry on enjoying the offerings of these care workers even after they had inevitably moved on to another job. I needed ownership of my family situation and as little stress as possible. Over time, I and those who cooked for us filled an attractive book with clear instructions for all the recipes my daughter and I enjoyed. Mealtimes became easier and more interesting, and out of what was often a difficult and unsettling situation grew a long-term project that came to be a self-published cookery book including foodie facts and folktales that I thought could encourage children to eat healthy food. I had spun a creative response from the straw of our enforced situation.

Another way I seize creative control when held hostage by my body, resentful of the same old ingredients of an ill life, is to reframe my situation as a reflection of a myth, folk tale or fantasy. This can help me accept my situation as something less unique to me, something imbued with archetypal themes.

Recently, in the midst of a health crash, when able to briefly swipe on my phone again, I posted a whimsical status on social media that both acknowledged how unwell I was and encouraged a more bearable way of experiencing the situation. 'I have appointed myself Queen of my world,' I wrote. 'I'm not a function-attending kind of queen. I reign from my bed-throne. Queens are known to delegate so there is no shame in having my meals brought to me, my consort wash me, and my crown shared around between more upright members of my realm.' My fantasy went on to explore the independent Wilderness Queen I'd rather be. For want of that reality I instead appointed friends and family my Wild Ambassadors to take me with them in spirit when enjoying their wild nature. I had found a way to reach out from my isolation, going so far as to hitch a virtual ride on their real-life adventures. My mum became my Wild Walks Ambassador. My sister, away on holiday, imagined me as a fairy stowed away in her pocket and, on her return, delivered holiday treats to my bed to make the experience more real for me. By embracing the fantasy, I turned some of the envy and sorrow that I had felt into inclusion. I had mustered a degree of sovereignty from within my recalcitrant body.

Beckett, a similarly ill friend reported from their own land, 'I am Ruler of Bed Island. We are a small island but known for our export of knitted goods.' Another, recovering from a recent trip away that her body was now paying the price for, sent a short video clip from a Scottish beach with the text, 'I accept the title of Wild Ambassador with pride.' Without leaving our beds we connected and I felt a little less left behind, a little more shimmering and seen.

Creating a role for yourself – artist, collator of recipes, sickness correspondent – or a whole-story metaphor may help you live better with your body's needs by providing a narrative that you can healthily embrace, rather than one foisted upon you that you yearn to resist. Instead of running from what will inevitably catch up with and damage us, we reclaim a degree of choice by turning to face it and re-naming, in our own terms, what is happening to us. Christine Miserandino harnessed the power of metaphor when inventing Spoon Theory to help healthy people better understand long-term illness. She came up with the idea when sitting at a table with cutlery on it while trying to convey her needs to a friend. The image came to her of a person starting their day with a fixed number of spoons, each of which represents one unit of energy and gets used up when performing any mental or physical task. While Spoon Theory doesn't appeal to everyone, it became so popular within the chronic illness community that being a Spoonie has become a unifying identity for many and the image of a spoon is now an icon for many with energy-limiting conditions.

Using the bones of your experience, imagine a character role for yourself in a story that you can live in with pride. It might not be the one you'd imagined for yourself but neither need you be relegated to a bit part. Even if the plotline is fixed you get to choose the tone and genre. Traditional fairy tales, artistic depictions, mythologies and personal folklore, created for and about yourself, all lend themselves to helping you feel more comfortable spinning the straw of your days into something more valued. Appendix 4: Metaphors and imagery to explore (page 325), contains a selection of ideas to get you started.

When straw doesn't shimmer like gold

Art needn't always be beautiful or uplifting. It is often a representation of the safe, routine and regular shaken up to something discombobulating, surprising or thought provoking. It is the same old colours or traditional images experienced in unexpected ways. It can be shocking, enlightening. We could even see our body as a piece of performance art, shaking things up and helping us to experience the world differently. Dan, a dancer who prefers not to disclose his disabling condition, has translated this idea to the stage. His theatrical movement pieces explore the balance of interdependence, care, varying levels of physical functionality and how to occupy a predominantly able-bodied world without feeling apologetic.

Our bodies and their unique responses to being alive become creative tools. We can draw up deep experiences, bringing them to the surface for examination and understanding. Channelled constructively, all emotions are valid hues on our palette. Anger, loss, grief, pain, fragile hope, pleasure, fear, defeat, acceptance. All can be expressed cathartically and aesthetically if we choose to use our creative powers in this way.

Of course, you don't have to use your creativity to exorcise suffering or assert yourself. You may prefer to turn to light relief. And you don't have to share your art with others if it's too personal. You create for yourself and that can be enough. Your creative self has no obligations to heal or educate. These are just potential side effects of expressing what you find within.

As you allow yourself to play creatively with your responses to difficulties, you may recognise an artistic style that has been so natural to you that you previously disregarded it. Maybe you considered it scruffy, non-descript, fussy or simplistic. To somebody else this may come across as free, fun, reminiscent of folk art, or expressive. This equally applies to the way we live. Our experiences and responses to them may not feel desirable, but the highlights and the threads of ourselves running throughout make the whole messy process worthwhile. If, either in daily living or our art, we can recognise satisfying qualities even in those things we don't like, we will become more able to expand our pockets of enjoyment and creativity.

> *Reclaim a sense of yourself as a creator of experience, as someone who constructively partners life's events, rather than a passive receptacle.*

Despite what our desire to achieve may tell us, perm-anent tangible output is not necessary for a fulfilling, creative life. You can ritually unravel old pieces of work as acknowledgment of how you may feel your life or personality has, to some extent, unravelled. And then create something anew. If your creative effort goes wrong, doesn't turn out how you anticipated, represents something painful to you, or is interrupted by health needs, it can be abandoned, resumed, revised, started all over again or completely discarded. You can leave it until you feel stronger or for when you have learnt new techniques or perspectives. Or you can move on from it entirely. Whether you do any of this out of necessity or as a conscious symbolic act, you are reclaiming a sense of yourself as a creator of experience, as someone who constructively partners life's events, rather than being a passive receptacle for struggle.

However you choose to express yourself, if your experience with chronic illness instigates a life lived more creatively, or inspires you to use your existing artistic urges to express a fresh perspective, then you have already begun to craft your path through your illness. You have already spun straw into gold.

Suggested therapeutic activity
Origami butterflies

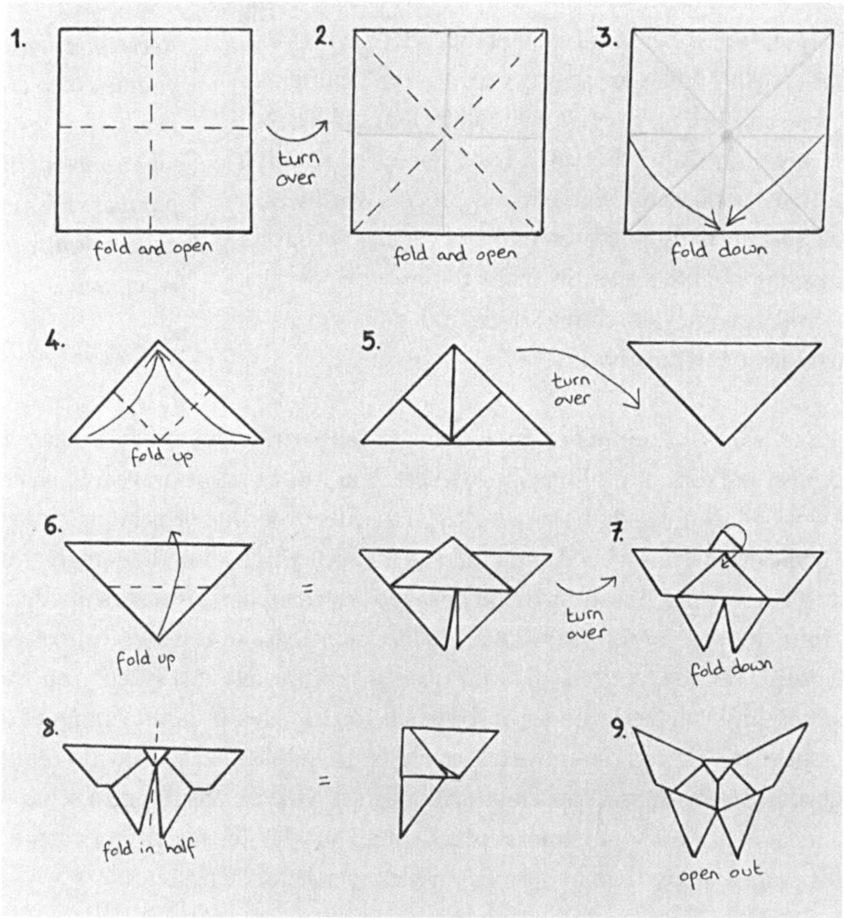

1. fold and open
2. turn over, fold and open
3. fold down
4. fold up
5. turn over
6. fold up
7. turn over, fold down
8. fold in half
9. open out

Chapter 10

Using discarded paper – old letters, medical information sheets, maps, paper bags, scraps of gift-wrap, unloved drawings, leaflets for events, etc. – symbolically enrich your relationship with the unwanted, the tired or the unattainable by creating your own version of the butterflies on the cover of this book.

1. With the right side facing up, fold a square of paper in half horizontally, pressing the fold firmly to make a sharp crease. Open the square back out. Repeat these actions folding vertically.
2. Turn the paper over so the other side is facing you and fold diagonally, pressing the crease, opening the paper out and repeating along the other diagonal.
3. Gently poke the centre of the square to encourage it to dip away from you and then take the centre point of the right edge and bring it down to the centre point of the bottom edge. The upper part of the square will collapse down with it. Repeat this action with the left edge, press the collapsed part flat, and you will now have a triangle.
4. Take hold of the upper layer of the right-hand corner and fold it upwards onto the top corner of the triangle, pressing the crease firmly with your fingers. Repeat with the left-hand corner.
5. Flip your almost-butterfly upside-down so that you are now looking at the other side of it, with the triangle pointing downwards.
6. Fold the upper layer of the bottom corner of the triangle upwards so that it extends a little beyond the centre of the opposite horizontal edge. This will cause the lower wings of the butterfly to separate a little.
7. Turn your butterfly over so you're looking at the other side. I like to leave the extended corner point sticking up beyond the edge as the head of the butterfly. If you would prefer to secure your butterfly a little more firmly, fold the extended corner over the edge to hold the layers together.
8. Fold your butterfly in half by bringing the top left and right wings up and together. Press this fold firmly.
9. Open the wings back out as far as you like and admire your butterfly.

Spinning gold from straw at a glance

- Without resorting to toxic positivity, we can choose to mine our situation for the hidden gold amongst the scratchy straw.
- Struggles such as isolation, limitation and boredom can inspire greater creativity.
- Illness and disability offer different perspectives from the status quo, resulting in diverse thought processes and representations.
- Difficult situations can be re-invented in our minds through fantastical story metaphors. This functions as both a coping mechanism and a launch pad for creative expression.
- Sometimes straw is just straw and this is okay. We don't always have to find gold or try to make straw something that it is not. Accepting this is a variant of gold in itself.

Chapter 11
Making room for creativity

Living day in, day out with the fallout of chronic illness, you may feel that all your expendable energy is used up on the essentials of living. Where is the joy, the momentary freedom, the melding of your psyche with a pleasurable pursuit? We don't want to simply survive. We want to thrive.

Illness may have forced you to step aside from a career, delegate responsibilities or turn down social events. Deprived of the usual distractions and diversions, frequently forced to withdraw from the outside world, newfound space opens up, inviting us to explore it creatively. Free time hovers impatiently, waiting to be filled. But we are navigating vastly limited energy reserves, sometimes overwhelming pain, and the practicalities of life may still feel all-consuming, with obligations eating up meagre energetic resources.

When our spare time does generously coincide with enough reduction in symptoms to allow us to experiment with our capabilities, that's when our inner creator can be encouraged out to play. Let us take some time now to consider how we can make more room for creativity to enrich our lives.

Simplify

First things first: simplify. Uncomplicate your life wherever you can. Employ any energy saving tips and tricks at your disposal, abandon what is unnecessary, accept help, and free yourself up for creative pleasures. It could be that gadgets around the home would ease household tasks or movements. Asking the council for a visit from an occupational therapist is one way of finding out what aids could be available to you, from an electric can opener to a shower seat, intercom system or stairlift.

When calculating what you can achieve in any given day, factor in time and energy for enjoyment. Energy is limited, symptoms reduce what you are able to engage in and enjoyment won't prioritise itself. There is no need to justify creative hobbies. This isn't a luxury to feel guilty about. Enjoying leisure activities may be more dependent on sacrifice for us than for healthy people, but we are no less deserving.

Accept help and free yourself up for creative pleasures.

So, simplify your life and make time for creative activity. Or to simply be still, letting fresh ideas swell, recede, rise again and arrive on the shores of your consciousness. Conserve your energy for what nurtures you. Then simplify your creative ideas so they are achievable. You can always build on these foundations later.

Practise declining, delegating and disappointing

People will behave with us how we allow them to so make it clear to family and friends that you will need to delegate, decline and disappoint at times. It's tempting to take on more than we should to keep others happy or get things done, even playing the martyr at times in the hope that others will spot our struggle and step in without needing to be asked. Tempting, but counterproductive.

Before over-exertion arises, state your limitations and where you could do with a bit more help. To maximise life with a chronic illness it is vital to take advantage of whatever opportunities for delegation are available. This doesn't make you lazy, nor does it imply that you're using your illness to your advantage. What it does mean is that you are learning to balance your needs, rather than following a preconceived concept of what you should be doing.

How you achieve this will depend on your circumstances. Perhaps you will ask for more engagement from friends and loved ones. Maybe employing a professional care worker, home help, PA or cleaner is the way forward, especially if you are eligible for financial assistance towards this from your local council. Looking at where, as a household, you could cut back on unnecessary expenditure may result in enough savings to either reduce work hours (if you or your partner are struggling to balance work with health needs) or to employ regular help or energy-saving devices. Or perhaps you would benefit from letting go of a perceived obligation that you persevere with at the expense of your physical and creative wellbeing.

Show yourself the care that you like to bestow on others by identifying your needs and requesting that they be taken into consideration. Others balance their responsibilities with leisure-time, and you have that right, too. It's just that your capacity for both is reduced and what may look to others like you indulging in relaxation is pre-emptive resting or post-exertion recuperation. Everyone needs to make time for play, even those of us busy apparently doing nothing.

> *Everyone needs to make time for play, even those of us busy apparently doing nothing.*

If this makes you feel guilty, remind yourself, as well as those you live with, that a happy you is more fun to be around than an overtired, grumpy with pain, creatively frustrated you. Prioritising your creative needs will therefore benefit others as well as you. Family members may, at first, feel disconcerted by your re-calibrated priorities. Dedicating some of your creative output to them or welcoming them to join you in your creative pursuits may be a way of getting them on board, helping them to feel included and still cared for.

Honesty with yourself

Our needs are more readily accommodated when we can address them with open awareness. Therefore, honesty about our limitations and where we may be haemorrhaging energy or exacerbating pain is paramount. Keeping life as uncomplicated as possible requires us to recognise our physical requirements and accept them. This doesn't mean resigning ourselves to them forever – just respecting them for now.

Have you fully acknowledged what you are giving your energy to, or do you try to live as 'normally' as possible, falling into a bemused heap at how unwell you feel with so little seemingly achieved? By acknowledging the reality of your situation, you will better learn to accommodate your body's needs without over-committing, making promises that will cause you physical or emotional stress, or having to entirely sacrifice creative fun.

Obstacles will arise, people will call on your energies, life needs attending to. There is no escaping that your health will be met with unexpected blows beyond your control. In the meantime, make the most of what you have by letting go of what doesn't require your attention. There will still be days, weeks, perhaps even months when you are unable to play creatively as you would like, but with careful energy management and selected priorities (not to mention a good relationship with the Fates) we can minimise the tools-down times and maximise our energy distribution.

An ill friend who was struggling with extreme levels of fatigue and pain, told me that there was no activity they could cut down on. They were already doing the bare minimum with nowhere left to conserve energy. The chat then revealed that, despite being housebound and in bed for much of the day, they were using precious energy to get themselves dressed. It can be hard to let go of standards and routines but liberating to forego activities that are not serving us. Getting dressed, washing, making the bed? Pfff! The world has plenty of people with those skills. Your energy levels and pain thresholds are limited so don't feel guilty about sometimes swapping mundane rituals in favour of what will bring you greater satisfaction.

On days when I know my energy levels will force me to choose between either getting dressed or a little creative work, I choose the latter. And I no longer feel odd about this. After a lifetime of illness, I've learnt to use what energy I have in the most constructive way I can. Sometimes this means throwing a shawl over my pyjamas, not letting any mirrors remind me of my unbrushed hair, piling up the supportive pillows and exploring a project.

It is important to be honest with yourself about how you may be mismanaging your physical resources when having fun. Pastimes that are restful for a healthy person could be sapping your energy without providing long-term reward. Watching television, playing online games, or scrolling through social media may all feel temporarily relaxing but your body is paying the cost whether you initially notice it or not. At times, playing a simple game on my phone may be all my concentration and weak hands can manage. Social media is where I often source artistic inspiration. But, if I'm not careful, the addictive nature of these pursuits can turn a rewarding few minutes into a habit that steals my available energy.

Ask yourself: when the day ends what will you be pleased to have spent time on? Different days will provide different answers so don't put pressure on yourself to always be productive. Just be aware of the choices you are making.

Some days you won't feel the freedom of choice. There will be times when your body will dictate the maximum it is willing to allow and that won't include your preferences. On the days when you can decide for yourself, do so consciously so that when you look back you are satisfied that you chose the most rewarding activities you could.

A dedicated space

One thing that turned around my ability to engage in creative pursuits was dedicating a personal space to arts and crafts. Hunting out materials and setting up equipment or tidying away a work in progress when strength is flagging consumes valuable energy. Sometimes just the thought of it would be too much for me.

After my daughter moved out, I had the luxury of turning her bedroom into a craft room. Now, when up to it, I wander into the next bedroom and pick something up that feels do-able. I can put it back down as it is, ready to be resumed in another brief flash of ability, without worrying about it being spread over the dining table or the act of tidying it away dismantling unsecured progress I may have made.

Many people don't have a spare room lying waiting to be designated with a purpose, but do try to claim some area purely for your creativity. It may be a cupboard that has been used as a dumping ground, an insulated shed in the garden, a corner of a living room, a desk in the exposed space under the stairs or a couple of storage baskets and trays of projects that slide out from under your bed, ready for action whenever you feel able to use them.

A pre-prepared physical space invites creativity. A pre-prepared physical space ritualistically and practically invites creativity. With one reach you can fiddle with fabric, play with the feel of pastels in your hand or enjoy the spectrum of paint tubes. It needn't be a permanent space. One year, Shannan, who lives with ME and the sound-sensitivity that often accompanies the condition, was struggling to cope with work taking place in her home. 'The floorboards had to be pulled up,' she recalls, 'and they were making one heck of a racket, which is why I hid in the garden in peace.' Not only did Shannan temporarily move into the garden, she created a dedicated sewing retreat for herself in a tent luxuriously filled with cushions and sewing materials.

If you are only well enough to manage 10 minutes of art or craft, you don't want to use up that time organising your workspace. Energy spent hunting for equipment that you know you own but can't find could have been used more effectively, so organise your creative space and materials in advance and prepare yourself to play as soon as your body next allows.

Suggested therapeutic activity
A creative opening ceremony
Design and create a dedicated space for your creativity. Whether this is as small as a lap tray with gathered materials or as dreamy as a whole craft room

at your disposal will depend on your circumstances. It might be a comfy chair with added cushions and blankets that is yours to curl up in with your creative expression journal, or a special pillow that you use to support yourself in bed and signify craft time. The important thing is that you have somewhere to indulge your creative side that you can turn to as regularly as possible.

Now it's time for the opening ceremony. If you live with other people, invite them to recognise this space and your intentions to use it as regularly as you are able. This will help you lend more weight to your creative side and can encourage those around you to realise what is important to you. Enjoy a special drink (or other edible treat) and raise a toast to your creative practice. Declare this space officially open!

Making room for creativity at a glance

- Set aside a little time and energy for creative pursuits, just as you would any other necessity.
- Be honest with yourself about where your energy is currently spent.
- Recognise your limitations and organise your life around these so that you forge space in your life for creative fun.
- Do less of the unnecessary.
- Be open about your needs and delegate chores wherever possible.
- Make yourself a dedicated space in your home for your creative hobbies. This can be as luxurious as a whole room or as small as a box of gathered materials. The only rules are that it is devoted to your creativity and easily accessible.
- Sometimes just one little change can instigate a whole different way of being.

Chapter 12
Getting the tension right

The overwhelming response I see in the chronic illness community to practising arts and crafts is how relaxing people find it. That's not to say frustration doesn't occur. Lizanne, a chronically ill visual artist experimenting with artistic doodling, sums it up: 'It's relaxing, if I'm not too hard on myself.'

When crafting flows well we enjoy the process and the effects that a relaxing hobby can have on our mental and physical symptoms, but only someone who has never strived to advance their skills would claim that arts and crafts are entirely tension-free. Tension, however, triggers your amygdala to move into a fear response. Not only is this in direct opposition to the relaxed state we want our struggling bodies to reside in, but it can cause creativity to freeze and play dead.

Feeling frustrated or despondent when our endeavours don't go to plan is occasionally inevitable, as is the physical strain that comes with new movements and concentration. Too much effort into mastering a skill, especially with a non-compliant body, will contraindicate any health benefits but we don't want to settle for less progress than we're capable of.

If difficulties are either panicking you back into a craft-scarce zone, or putting your body out of action, they have become counterproductive. Just as in knitting and crochet, where there is a perfect tension to be found somewhere between too tight and too loose, so there is that sweet spot between pushing yourself too hard and giving up too soon.

So, how do we settle into that desired tension between slackness and stress?

Beginning to relax

At the beginning of a learning curve the frustration of not being able to achieve what expectations promised can escalate. If not seen in perspective, such setbacks can put some people off creating at all. This is a shame as these are often temporary difficulties, encountered by many before us who have ended up surprising and impressing themselves.

While learning a new technique, muscles and tendons may rebel against the unusual moves you're asking of them. To minimise this as much as possible, make a conscious effort to relax into your actions and start with very short practice sessions. Unsure of how to proceed with a new activity, or uncertain as to whether we're doing it correctly, we tend to scrutinise our work, hunching over with squinted eyes. As we become more familiar with our new hobby, these strains will lessen. In the meantime, scan your body mentally for any tension you can release or a more relaxed posture you can adopt. Keep dropping your shoulders and slackening your jaw.

Art and craft virgins may find that their first choice is causing frustration they need not be encumbered with if they investigate a different style or another craft altogether. Resist falling into the trap of assuming that inability to work in one genre implies a lack of creative ability altogether. It can take time to find your creative niche. But before abandoning what threaten to be dead ends, first consider how any problems could be side-stepped or whether you may simply have excessive expectations of yourself. We might just need a little advice or constructive guidance. 'The fingers-and-thumbs phase is part of the standard learning process' and 'It does get more calming' are just two examples of encouragement I was offered by other chronically ill crafters when I first attempted crochet.

It can take time to find your creative niche. Rather than being scared off, be curious about the creative process.

Feeling clueless when you encounter something new is natural. Rather than being scared off, be curious about the creative process.

The brain's neurotransmitter when encountering curiosity is dopamine and, when released in generous quantities, dopamine provides us with a sense of pleasure and reward. The more curiosity you can summon, as opposed to frustration or defeatism, the happier you will feel.

Admittedly, crochet and I still aren't best of friends, but that's fine. I achieved my goal of making something simple and I recognised that I'm more at home with knitting needles than a crochet hook. Where I used to get wound up about my clumsy attempts, I now rest more peacefully in the knowledge that we can't all be good at everything. Which leads us nicely on to…

Dropping pressure

Current obstacles may feel like hurdles too high for you to jump, but creativity reminds us that if we can't leap then perhaps we can limbo underneath them. Lean back from persistent struggle and shimmy into a variant that works better for you. While creativity might turn the music up, eager for a good limbo (to stretch this metaphor a little further), chronic illness often just prefers a quiet lie down, opening its eyes only intermittently to peek beyond the hurdle. So, take a rest and see what options come to mind as you examine the lie of the land. Perhaps you can just lower the bar?

However you choose to proceed – under, over, around; now or later – take care not to squander precious energy resources on self-inflicted stress. Be wary of setting yourself up for failure by wanting to emulate healthy artists with heaps of practice under their belt. You are working within the confines of physical limitations beyond your control, so form realistic goals. 'I have found it relaxing having *no* goals or expectations,' says one member of an online group when sharing her painted representation of a flower border. Meanwhile, Melissa, who was a professional artist and art teacher before developing chronic illness, has this to say about reducing the tension that can arise from a deficit of energy or inspiration to create what she used to: 'I don't have to create a masterpiece. I stick to something easy, sometimes cutting out images for collage or doing an abstract drawing that means nothing at first. An adult colouring-book can be relaxing. Even a paint-by-numbers kit can get my juices flowing. If I have the energy to come back the next day or next week, I try to put things together. It is hard to accept that I cannot be as productive as before, but doing something is better than nothing for me.'

Maintain a healthy sense of sustainability by freeing yourself from pressure.

Find where you can maintain a healthy sense of sustainability, by freeing yourself from unnecessary pressure, resting when you need to, giving yourself permission to take as long on a project as your body requires, and choosing to create whatever feels achievable for you.

Self-awareness

Becoming more aware of any mental, emotional or physical stress being held isn't always easy, especially if you are habituated to tight muscles and other symptoms associated with tension in either your body or mind. It can help to let the work you are creating educate and guide you in this matter. Are you unintentionally creating very small or irregular embroidery stitches? Is your knitting or crochet too tight or uneven? Are your pencil marks excessively heavy or stilted? These outcomes can indicate that you are experiencing stress or anxiety that you may not be consciously aware of.

Relax and gently endeavour to loosen or calmly regulate your hand movements. This in turn can have a positive effect on your internal state. Breathe out an extended exhalation, accept that you feel tense and access your personal calm-triggers. These could be looking out of the window at a favourite tree, stroking a pet, listening to music, taking time out to laugh at a comedy programme, meditating, having a nap or reciting an affirmation that encourages calm strength.

Positive self-talk can help outweigh the negative thoughts that arise when things don't go to plan. Talking in the second person, as if encouraging someone else, has been shown to be most effective at this, resulting in lower levels of upset and greater objectivity about the difficulty being encountered. 'Come on, Germaine, you can do this,' I will often say out loud, as well as: 'Well done, you!'

Be gentle with yourself and as kind as you would to somebody else who is struggling. Criticising and getting cross with yourself or your materials feels like a release of tension in the moment (and, heaven knows, I've fallen into that trap) but the stress hormones released will likely be detrimental to your physical and emotional wellbeing in the long run. They also risk causing any tentative creativity to retreat like a chastised child. Talk to yourself encouragingly and acceptingly, aware of when you are enjoying yourself enough to continue and when a different strategy is called for.

Finding the right tension for you…

To return to the analogy of tension in yarn work: tight stitches in amigurumi crochet make for compact toys whose stuffing stays firmly in place, whereas a loose tension in knitting can enhance an open-weave lacy effect. Both serve a purpose. Similarly, tight control when drawing creates a distinctive effect that is no better nor worse than the free, energetic effect of a looser rein on the pencil.

When it comes to personal tension, weigh up for yourself whether to go with the tighter efforts of a tricky learning curve or to ease up on yourself and give another project a go instead. A little tension may feel invigorating for those who revel in a challenge, while others may find a more laid-back approach is what their mind and body require. It is up to you to decide which works best for you at any given time.

Perhaps your current project is not appropriate for you, or the project is manageable but your approach to it needs a little adjustment. Maybe it is a challenge that you want to persevere with but need a temporary break from.

Stimulating some quick hits of dopamine with a simple speedy make may be what you need right now. Having an easy, relaxing project on the go at the same time as a more focused one will allow you to swap between the two, maintaining your engagement with crafting while spreading out any physical or mental effort.

...So the fun can flow free

Should you find craft-related tensions are outweighing the pleasures, consider your relationship with your chosen activity. Is it that the physical actions are causing discomfort? Are you dissatisfied with what you produce? Seek to alter your materials, posture, technique or expectations so you can relax more deeply into the pleasurable sensations of your craft. Allow a piece to develop its own character – even if that strays from how you originally envisaged it – and have fun. The aim here is simply to create therapeutic-grade entertainment.

The aim is to create therapeutic-grade entertainment.

It can be helpful to establish whether the tension of your efforts would benefit from being tightened or slackened to enhance your enjoyment. If the project is either too difficult or too easy, you could be denying yourself the much sought-after experience of flow state.

Flow state refers to those moments when we are partaking in an activity and time seems to disappear. We are in the zone and the rest of the world temporarily drops away. Ideas, motivation and focus abound. Flow state is most likely to occur when the tension between ease and difficulty in what we are doing hits our personal sweet spot. Too easy and tedium may be experienced, too difficult and frustration occurs. That space where we are striving with a degree of effort but without excess struggle – that is where the joy of flow state resides. Look to find this balance whenever you and your creativity play together.

According to preliminary research, the brain uses slightly less energy to achieve tasks when in a flow state than normally. For those who find cognitive engagement physically draining, this is great news. Less energy expenditure means more opportunity to indulge in fun.

Suggested creative exercise
Pressure points

Grab a sheet of plain paper and a pencil. Now doodle, draw, practice shading, write freely or copy out a loved verse. It doesn't matter what you do – but do it firmly. Apply pressure with the pencil. Now repeat the action but, this time, gently. Use a light touch and see if your body's reaction, your mind's response or the results on the paper differ. Experiment with a variety of different pressures and observe the effects.

Now consider how this could be applied to your creative hobbies. Try something a little lighter to partake in than you might usually, and then something a little harder, just to test your ultimate comfort zone and how these different efforts affect you. Do you want to continue with either of these directions or return to where you were before? Perhaps your choice will vary day to day.

Getting the tension right at a glance

- Be patient with yourself when learning a new craft. Take it slowly, giving your body and brain time to settle in.
- If one craft is proving continuously stressful, try another.
- Let go of expectations about the quality of your work. Enjoy the process.
- Make your self-talk encouraging, not critical.
- Regularly relax any tense muscles.
- Find balance between too easy and too difficult and you are more likely to settle into 'flow state' where anything other than the experience at hand drops away into insignificance.

Chapter 13
Stopping up the energy leaks

Those of us with chronic illness must monitor our energy with extra care. Awareness of where our reserves leak away gives us more likelihood of achieving our desires. Our body may hold the upper hand, but it is up to us to make the most of what we do have control over.

Your condition will mean that your needs are unique to you. Pay attention to what affects your health, both positively and negatively, and make the effort to do what best serves you. So many times I have thought, 'I'll be fine. I'm just doing this for a moment' only to find myself suffering afterwards because I ignored either the warning signs from my body or knowledge gained from past experiences.

Never ignore discomfort that you can remedy. It may seem stoic or easier than getting up and adjusting your surroundings or posture, but it piles extra strain on an already struggling body. If you are chronically ill, presume that you will only be fine if you take good precautions and best measures to achieve your long-term goals.

I invested in a smartwatch that monitors my heartrate, stress level and 'body battery'. It allows me to recognise what activities are putting my body under extra duress that I may not otherwise have recognised until the after-effects kick in. However, such equipment doesn't tell you how to reduce the normal stresses that a clinically unwell body over-reacts to, often after a misleading delay. It is simply a tool to increase awareness of when a rest could be beneficial, when you may be safe to expend a little creative energy, and whether you could benefit from employing some of the following tips.

Paying attention to your senses

Are you warm enough? Too hot? We may not be able to fully control a wonky inner thermostat or circulatory system, but adjusting the surrounding temperature via heating, an electric fan or open windows are simple ways to reduce how hard your body works to maintain homeostasis. If you get cold easily but find the weight of thick jumpers impedes your movements, then consider thin thermal underwear, lap blankets, fingerless gloves, a hot water bottle or electric heat pad to increase body temperature without hampering your arms. These are also cheaper options than heating the whole home, leaving more financial resources for craft materials!

Think about the lighting in your chosen work area. Is it bright enough to avoid eyestrain while being as close to natural light as possible? The glare from overly bright bulbs or screens takes its toll on our bodies even if we are unaware of it in the moment.

Could unnecessary noise or extraneous visual stimuli be distracting or draining you? Sensory overload saps energy, sometimes without us even noticing at the time. Reducing what your brain is having to process can free up more energy for your creative endeavours, so if you routinely keep the television on or listen to music then consider turning these off or switching to less stimulating playlists or programmes. Of course, you may find lively music invigorates and motivates you. Just take care to recognise how it affects you, both in the short and long term.

If surrounding sounds beyond your control are sapping your energy and increasing unpleasant symptoms, noise reduction ear plugs (such as ear loops that allow you to hear localised sounds while softening other noises) or ear defenders may be worth considering. Alternatively, listening to white noise or recordings of nature sounds may dampen intrusive sounds.

And what about hunger and thirst? I can find that just one oatcake, a couple of dried apricots or a handful of nuts can be enough of a remedy when my blood sugar levels start to drop, so take a moment to consider whether you could benefit from a small, healthy snack or a drink. Being hydrated is especially important for those with low blood volume, which can be a feature of ME/CFS and PoTS.

Posture and muscle use

Is your chair the right height for your worktable, or your tray the right height over your lap? I have sent myself into a health crash before now just by sitting slightly too low at a table, unconsciously hunching my shoulders to raise my arms. This extra muscle use, leading to painfully weak muscles as well as increased generalised fatigue, was entirely avoidable if I had paid attention to how I was sitting.

Placing a cushion in the small of your back when sitting upright helps your spine to maintain its natural conformation, thus keeping the rest of the body happier. An ergonomic seat-cushion, meditation cushion or a rolled-up towel can also help to achieve this. However, remember to remain comfortably flexible rather than fixed to one position, which in itself can drain energy.

In my teens, when being taught how better to manage my health, I was told by a rare professional who understood my condition, 'When standing see if you could be sitting. When sitting see if you could be lying.' Unless it is alleviating pain or otherwise benefiting your body, why use energy in standing at an easel or dressmaker's dummy, for example, when you could sit on a stool? And why sit up unaided when an appropriately cushioned or ergonomic chair could be taking some strain off your core muscles? If being upright, even propped against pillows, puts strain on your muscular or circulatory system then investigate ways of creating while lying down, or at least semi-prone, perhaps with an angled lap tray or over-bed table. Simply having your legs raised can reduce the effort your body has to make if blood flow is compromised, perhaps by orthostatic intolerance.

Even seemingly small amounts of muscle use can cause disproportionate levels of pain, fatigue, tremors, post-exertional malaise and other symptoms for the chronically ill creator. One way to help minimise this is to rest your arms, instead of holding them aloft, wherever possible. Allowing your elbows to be close to your body rather than held out at the sides is another small postural difference that can have a larger impact on energy usage than you may realise. Diverting your energy expenditure away from such minutiae as supporting your own musculature frees it up for more creative exertions. Cushions, neck pillows, stretch bandages, a neck brace and whatever else provides you with a little extra strength, stability and conserved energy are all worth considering.

Allowing your elbows to be close to your body rather than held out at the sides can have a larger impact on energy usage than you may realise.

Get into the habit of regularly checking whether you are tensing or using any muscles unnecessarily. Are you leaning forward over your work when you could be resting against support or maintaining a healthier posture? Mentally scan your whole body for anywhere that could benefit from instant relaxation. Shoulders, eyes and jaw are key areas to pay attention to, as well as your pelvic floor and stomach if you are prone to stress when trying to achieve something challenging.

Heat pads (sometimes best alternated with ice packs) are invaluable for many in relaxing muscles and soothing pain that we can unwittingly tense against. If you hold yourself awkwardly due to inflammatory pain, ice packs can help to reduce this, leaving you more able to sit in a way that doesn't create problems of its own.

Consider also whether glasses may reduce any potential eye-strain. I find that over-using my eye muscles, through reading or close-up work, leads to worsened dizziness, nausea, headaches, migraine, neck and spinal pain. Never underestimate the knock-on effects of using the tiny muscles that are so integral to everyday life that we forget we're employing them.

Chapter 13

Stretch yourself…

I still find it surprising how much energy my body consumes just by maintaining a static, yet unnatural position. Pay attention to how you are holding your body and, if your activity doesn't allow you to switch into a more natural position, stave off any potential problems with regular compensatory stretches, shoulder rolls and head movements. Even with very limited mobility, muscles that have been in one position, or engaged in repetitive actions, usually benefit from any gentle, balancing stretching you can safely manage within the limitations of your condition, especially just after or during a crafting session.

Make a point of letting your shoulders drop, shaking out your arms and wiggling your fingers. Move your head and rotate your neck. When focusing your eyes on close-up work, take regular momentary breaks to close your eyes or soften your gaze to a far-off horizon or the furthest edge of the room. Release any tension that could result in a deeper slide into exhausting symptoms.

> *Muscles that have been in one position, or engaged in repetitive actions, usually benefit from gentle stretching.*

Carson Demers has forged a name for himself as the Ergonomic Knitter. He recommends stretching your fingers and hands out wide from an initial fist shape to release tightened or painful forearms and tendonitis. He also suggests looking up regularly from your work so that your neck isn't continuously bent down. When you do find yourself working with your head down, every so often tuck in your chin by gliding your head backwards to get as many double chins as possible and then release. Demers maintains that repeating this a couple of times in a row helps to strengthen the neck.

If you have been advised to follow physiotherapy exercises, be sure to do these as often as your body responds well to. Put your body in the best possible condition for achieving your goals. Some people find gentle yoga or pilates helpful for maintaining the scope of what they can achieve and releasing physical tension that is further sapping their energy. For those of us with extremely limited energy, just a minute or two of chair or bed yoga may be beneficial. An internet search will reward you with links to yoga routines or other appropriate stretches.

…And relax

When stressed, our heart rate increases, muscles tense and energy is run through at an alarming rate. Additionally, a stressed brain can interpret sensations as more painful than when calm. Whenever you find yourself learning a new technique, absorbed in a tricky process, rushing to finish something or holding your body uncomfortably, take a moment to check your subconscious stress level and to consciously relax. Soften your forehead, loosen your jaw, drop those shoulders, relax your stomach and exhale. Take any self-imposed pressure off yourself, rather than adding ammunition to your illness's armoury. Close your eyes and take a rest, just for a few seconds… minutes… or longer. As long as you need.

Similarly, being eager, excited or jubilant can over-stimulate a fragile body, burning up more energy reserves than the enjoyable feelings in the moment would lead you to believe. That's not to say we can't indulge and revel in the moment, but we must help our body recalibrate to a state of calm as soon as possible with whatever tried-and-trusted relaxation methods work for us.

Cyclic sighing (or cyclic breathing) is a breathwork technique that is particularly good at activating the parasympathetic nervous system, which lowers the heart rate and switches the body into a state of greater relaxation. Any time you feel you could benefit from it, take a comfortably deep breath in through your nose, so your abdomen moves out, pause for a moment before inhaling further to fully fill your lungs, and then exhale very slowly through an almost closed mouth (as if blowing through a straw) to prolong the outbreath for as long as is comfortable. When practising this technique, my exhalations tend to last for two to three times as long as my full inhalation. It is recommended that you repeat this for five minutes, although I have at times found that just a few of these breaths can, according to the stress score on my smart watch, bring me greater relaxation. It has its limits, having no effect on the stress that digesting heavy food or coping with extreme post-exertional malaise puts on my system, but it is a constructive tool that has been shown to help the sympathetic nervous system to settle, as well as helping alleviate anxiety.

Suggested therapeutic activity

Body scan

Close your eyes and mentally observe your body. Beginning with either your toes or the top of your head, work your way throughout your body, tuning in to how all parts are feeling. Is anywhere tense? If so, consciously relax those muscles. Do any specific symptoms that you've been ignoring need attending to? Could you make yourself more comfortable in any small way? Scan your whole body and respond appropriately to anything you notice. If you feel any discomfort that is beyond your control, rather than trying to change it, breathe into it, summon a sense of compassion for this part of you and allow your mind to consider what that body part might more broadly benefit from.

Stopping up the energy leaks at a glance

- Pain and tension use up energy. Respond appropriately to these, rather than trying to ignore them.
- Take measures against excess sounds, or light that is too bright or too dim.
- Maintain a comfortable body temperature.
- Ensure your body is well supported.
- Regularly stretch and change positions.
- Relax eye muscles by periodically gazing into the far distance.
- Breathe calmly, with the emphasis placed on exhalations.
- Use any tools or aids that can assist you. Refer to your chosen style of craft in Chapter 17: Create-ability, in Part 4, for suggestions.

Chapter 14
From pushing to pacing

How often have you yearned for more than your body can safely maintain? It's so tempting to push through symptoms, or embark on a creative adventure, despite knowing that such actions may well incur debilitating delayed reactions. After all, who wants to face the prospect of stopping what they enjoy, saying 'No, not now; maybe never'?

Ignoring our body's warning signs may achieve a burst of productivity in the short term but risks being severely detrimental down the line. I have known it drive me into a reduced level of living from which I looked longingly back to the stage I had previously been bemoaning. From that vantage point I invariably wish I'd paced better.

But sometimes temptation beckons a little too urgently. Even the smallest immersion in creativity can be a vital antidote to feeling trapped by illness, and so pushing in that direction feels like the right move. Living with clinical levels of fatigue and discomfort means that at times we force ourselves through pain and exhaustion to partake in things that help us feel wilfully alive.

We will best maximise our ability to engage with creative fun if we balance the (sometimes necessary) desire to push ourselves with the essential art of pacing our energy. Booming and busting, highs and crashes – however you refer to this cycle of over-exertion followed by extended recovery time, it results in more pain and frustration in the long run than if you had stopped a little sooner to give your body some time out. It's not easy, I know. (I really, really do!) Resentment of your situation is a real risk that can lead to you throwing your hands up in the air and chucking caution to the wind, only to berate yourself later when your body doles out the consequences.

Learning to pace my energy was forced upon me when, some 30 years ago, I ignored how severely unwell I really was and pushed myself into a previously undiscovered depth of my condition that I have never fully emerged from. Until I had no other choice, I balked at the idea of resting ahead of incapacitation. I wanted to get as much out of life as possible and couldn't accept that, by pushing myself, I was approaching a precipice that I was to fall over quite unceremoniously. I still find that frustration, impatience and boredom when resting, as well as enjoyment of what I'm involved in when more able, can propel me into unwise activity if I'm not careful, but I now live within wiser parameters.

When and when not to push yourself

Some days you *will* have to push yourself to get started. You may be acutely aware of the continuous pain, discomfort or fatigue that prevents you from feeling properly up to doing anything beyond essential self-care, but you know that this is the status quo for you and if you always acted on how you physically felt you'd never do anything creative. By giving something a go, a little adrenaline may flow, bringing with it some natural pain relief and tucked away reserves of energy. Even without adrenaline, if you start to enjoy yourself and slip into pleasant thoughts and motion, pain sometimes recedes from the forefront of awareness for a while.

This is a very delicate balancing act. There is a price to pay for running on adrenaline, so we learn to borrow it judiciously, prepared to pay up when our body demands repayment, sometimes with extortionate interest fees.

Our symptoms are often warning signals that we ignore at our peril. While we don't want to let our health set all the rules of living (succumbing to a life of nothing but illness rarely feels an acceptable option), living within our boundaries is necessary if the illness isn't to gain complete control. We make considered demands of our body, but we also surrender to our condition's requirements in order to negotiate a working relationship with it, neither giving up in the face of illness nor enacting a constant battle with it. By listening to and cooperating with our symptoms we become more amicable bedfellows with our condition.

So, sometimes our body needs a little encouragement out of a slump but sometimes it needs extended and intensive rest and recuperation. At times, the unpalatable after-effects of using energy that wasn't really at our disposal is outweighed by the sense of expression and achievement we attained by pushing ourselves. At other times we are better off letting our body build its energy reserves, rather than worsening our symptoms or initiating a long and tedious relapse. It is for us, with our personal experience of our illness, to make the best choices we can.

The really tricky times come when we know we can push a bit, and enjoy being in the flow of creativity, but must remain mindful of stopping while the going is good. Just because we have been able, for a while, to keep going regardless of our symptoms, does not mean we should continue to do so. Would you encourage a marathon runner to repeat the circuit the moment they reach the finish line? Remember the marathon that your body perceives when performing activities others can do without concern.

One way to assess your capability is to pay attention to the cycle your body is currently in. If you have been pushing yourself for a little while or have been exposed to stressors (a virus, hormone fluctuations, worry, or positive stress like being excited about some good news or impending event) then take extra care to pace your energy with careful consideration.

If you are just coming out of a health dip, you will be working on limited energy reserves and your newfound increase of energy or reduction in symptoms could be a thin layer over a deep chasm. Tread carefully, lighten the load by laying down your craft tools and resting horizontally when you can and give this new ground time to build up its layers of stability. Even then, we are in precarious territory and must always be mindful of potential sinkholes beneath us. That's just the way it is with chronic illness.

While pushing our physical and cognitive energy too far leaves us depleted and without the resources to regulate our emotions as we'd like, pushing our creativity can also be counterproductive. Just like trying hard to remember a forgotten word utilises the wrong part of the brain for recollection, forcing creativity puts us in a different mindset from the one needed for ideas to flow. However, there are times when a little extra effort can be rewarding. So, push a little, pace a lot and be willing to change the rhythm as your body requests.

Pacing your learning

If you are discovering a new craft, treading this fine line between pushing and pacing can have additional difficulties. In the first stages of learning you may feel that if you don't persevere until you've got the hang of it you will never master the moves. In this case, it might be that a little extra pushing is worth the payback your body will endure. However, beware of being tricked by a doubtful or over-eager mind that wants you to do more in one session than is wise.

Beware of an over-eager mind that wants you to do more in one session than is wise.

When acquiring a new skill, you are using your body and brain in new ways. This is tiring but will become easier as you relax into the process and build up habitual memory. Don't be overly concerned if at first your body reacts in a way that leads you to believe your chosen craft is beyond your reach. Rest and come back to it, for micro-sessions, later. Even muscles that are affected negatively by exercise can, to a degree, become a little happier with new movements if they are eased in very gently over time. And even sparse and sporadic practice can lead eventually to satisfying results.

Chapter 14

Give yourself short, monitored, time-slots to push through difficulties and then plenty of time to rest and recover. By repeating this process you will discover, within safely regulated boundaries, whether you can persevere without too many repercussions and how well your body can adjust to what you're asking of it. Perhaps it can't tolerate this activity; maybe it needs you to adapt how you engage in it; or simply to reduce your practice time to smaller sessions. Hopefully you'll find yourself building up to a little more immersion as time goes by. To invite a greater chance of picking up your chosen endeavour again sooner rather than later, pace yourself by resting often and keep a check on that desire to push for instant results.

Take these breaks before it feels absolutely necessary and you have a stronger likelihood of preventing yourself from being incapacitated by enforced, lengthy recovery. Too long a gap between instalments in the beginning stages will hinder what you retain and can thus build upon, so use short sessions to maximise the regularity with which you are able to return to your craft and maintain an encouraging momentum. The alternative is to push yourself hard enough to make giant initial leaps only to spend so much time in physical recovery that you can't consolidate what you've learnt.

Before you start to resent the breaks your illness forces you to take from practising your new craft, bear in mind that anyone learning something new benefits from regular pauses to process the information being fed to it. The brain doesn't retain information through binge-learning but via regular educational instalments. Pacing the path of learning with sleep in between sessions enables healthy and ill people alike to come back to the task primed for greater improvement than if they'd pushed through in one mammoth session. Whatever your health, giving your body and brain the space to accommodate the development you're asking of them may prove more productive than impatiently pushing yourself.

Finding your own pace

So, it's a given that expressing your creative side would enhance your life and keep some of the illness blues at bay, but your situation seems to prohibit immersion in activity. Don't despair! Pushing-and-pacing is all about personal balance, and the continuation of your crafting practice can be approached like a personalised prescription in which small doses remain the safest way to avoid side effects. You may wish you could take a larger dose, and in time you may increase it, but it's crucial to recognise how much activity is sustainable before risking more repercussions than were bargained for. Just as taking medication is best overseen by a pharmacist or doctor, carers and understanding family members can be invaluable for helping us to notice when we require a dose of our chosen creative medicine and when we need to abstain.

No engagement, no matter how short, is insignificant. I know people who are only able to crochet for five to 10 minutes at a go. Over time, they produce impressive work. Others can progressively increase their session lengths until they reach a personal plateau. Some plateaux turn out to be launch pads for future advances; others may be your pinnacle. Either way, use careful time management to keep the chances of a steady path in your favour.

One body may struggle with particular physical movements while another cannot tolerate focused concentration. You may find that you have different boundaries for different activities. Perhaps you have difficulty enduring specific combinations? Do these vary depending on other factors influencing your health at any given time? Observe how you cope with different activities and any delayed reactions they may incur. Accept with compassion where your body struggles. This brings you closer to discovering how to integrate your needs with your desires, rather than pushing yourself into an all-or-nothing situation.

To respond appropriately to your health, you first need to be able to under-

Chapter 14

stand its language. I always thought my body was sending crazily mixed messages until I learned what was going on behind the scenes. I couldn't understand why I often felt worse in the short term when I rested but better in the long term. Why, when I found it hardest to lie still, twitching agitatedly with a buzzing urge to be active, did I, given perseverance, fall into deep, clearly beneficial, sleep? What was my body playing at, making the remedy so hard to swallow? How was I to listen to my body when it spoke only in riddles?

In my case, learning how an over-active sympathetic nervous system was reacting to radically reduced energy levels taught me why some of the physical phenomena felt counter-intuitive. I now realise that feeling energised to the point of racing thoughts and a fizzing sensation in my veins is not a sign that I should be getting stuck into a high-energy craft project, no matter how right it feels in the moment.

Quite the reverse.

I have learnt to recognise the pumped-up alarm calls of a system under great strain for what they are. If my skin has been pallid, pain troublesome and my muscles unresponsive to my will, but forced activity fires me up to rosy-cheeked ability, this is not a good sign. It is often seen by onlookers as proof that I just needed stimulation but is, in fact, my body going into emergency mode, pulling out all the stops to get me through the moment before leaving me worse than before.

So, listen not just to the momentary sensations but to their underlying message. Pay attention, learn about the workings of your condition, and time will teach what your body is requesting of you. There is a theory that if you always wait until your body is screaming at you to take a break, your brain will deduce that it must send powerful signals to force you to take care of yourself. By doing right by your personal needs before the pain or fatigue becomes intolerable, you not only keep some energy reserves in store, and reduce the likelihood of a symptom flare, but (so the theory goes) your brain learns to trust you to look after yourself without requiring such severe warning signs.

One factor that enabled me to run the magazine I mentioned in Chapter 7: Creating purpose (page 77), was my recognition of my limited pace of work. A magazine was a canny idea for someone with limited energy as it could be filled with other people's articles and illustrations, but I knew I couldn't work on it regularly enough to distribute it as frequently as most periodicals. Realistically, I could only manage two issues a year. So that's what I did. I calculated my achievable expectations and, thanks to not setting my sights too high or conforming to typical practice, I succeeded in keeping my dream afloat. One year, my health necessitated a delayed issue release. An explanatory email was sent to shops and subscribers, and nobody minded. My pace was entirely acceptable.

I had to pace my life around this project accordingly: leisure reading was sacrificed so that my eyes could cope with editing, and other creative pursuits went by the wayside for the magazine's lifespan.

Learning to partake of fun in small, regular doses and downing tools when creative energy is still flowing isn't easy, especially when you know others are crafting for hours on end, but this isn't a competition. You will make progress in your own time. You will also obtain a greater sense of satisfaction from being able to craft briefly but regularly than from overworking and crashing. Lior has certainly found this to be the case: 'I pick up the ukulele for one song a day, then stop unless I'm having a particularly good day. I'll dance to one song. I'll draw for a few minutes at a time. It's sustainable. I also log in a bullet journal whether I've been able to do a few minutes of these various things I value. It means that I see the data on the page, the proof that I am creating. Over time I've really let go of it not being of huge quantity or even quality. For now, it's just about direction. I'm going in the

> *You will get better at pacing the more you practise it and feel the reward of having taken good care of yourself.*

right direction, creating what I can, and that's all that can be asked of anyone.'

You get to choose your own expectations of your creativity and your life's direction with this condition. Take time to consciously decide what those expectations are rather than following where peers, family or old preconceptions may have been misguidedly leading you.

We all know that practice makes perfect. You will get better at pacing the more you practise it and feel the reward of having taken good care of yourself. As for your craft, you cannot practise that if you are suffering more than usually from having pushed yourself too much the day or week before. One large attempt that sets your body back is dispiriting so, instead, think of the bigger picture and allow multiple small attempts to build upon each other.

It's all about the timing

Cutting your enjoyment short when you feel able to continue, or even when the pain is intense but you really want to finish what you're doing, is incredibly hard. It's like being sent to bed on a summer evening when you were young and could hear neighbourhood children still playing outside.

I struggle with knowing when to stop. My condition manifests its reactions to exertion anything from immediately to 72 hours after the event, as well as producing emergency adrenaline that masks pain and depleted energy. Additionally, difficulty with both starting and stopping activities can be a neurological symptom of some conditions. Once I have mustered up the energy to get going on a project, my body and mind lock into wanting to continue. I know from experience the danger of doing too much but how much easier it is to convince myself that this time I'll be fine to carry on just a teeny bit longer. And longer. And… oops, I overdid it again.

My advice for combating this is a timer. Whether art-ing, crafting or browsing online for inspiration and information, use your timer to encourage yourself to stay within a safe energy-expenditure range. In the past I have used a cheap-and-cheerful wind-up cat timer that would twist to any time span up to an hour, ticking away reliably. Having a fun, feline-shaped timer helped me perceive the buzzing of the alarm more as a gentle paw on my lap, encouraging me to pause for a cosy cat-nap, than as an enforced disability aid nagging me to halt my fun. I now prefer the gentle vibration on my wrist of a smart-watch timer. If you opt for a digital timer, always check that you've set it correctly before entrusting yourself to its timekeeping. Several times I've set mine only to realise, too late when my crafting session seemed to have lasted enjoyably longer than usual, that I selected the wrong time or forgot to press 'start'.

I have a consistent habit of wanting to spend far longer on what I'm engaged in than the time I've allotted for myself. I've found that setting my timer for a shorter duration than I know I can actually allow myself provides that great feeling of being given extra time when I re-set it, if I'm in full flow or at a crucial problem-solving moment.

Just like a child needing a five-minute warning before having to tidy away their toys, I always require a little buffer time for tying up loose ends or winding down before my final call to set down tools. I wholly recommend factoring this in when choosing how long to set your timer for and always setting it for five minutes less than the duration you initially decided on. And never ever tell yourself, 'This will only take another five minutes', without resetting your timer or using a snooze function so that you are alerted when your time's really up. If the 'five minutes' in your house are like the ones that live in mine, you'll find they readily transform into time warps when not kept a careful eye on.

Another way of using a timer that many find helpful, if they don't need to be quite so strict about only working for a prescribed quantity of time, is the pomodoro technique. Recommended as a way of maximising productivity, it is also employed by some in the chronic illness community to remind them to take regular rest breaks. In fact, the author Susanna Clarke used this technique when writing her novel *Piranesei*. The idea is that you work for 25 minutes at a time, with five-minute breaks in between. Every fifth break should be a longer rest, lasting for between 15 and 30 minutes. While this is easy enough to implement with any timer, pomodoro and productivity apps are widely available.

For some, the idea of a timer may seem too regimented, but there are other ways to keep track of your energy expenditure. If you craft while watching television or listening to radio programmes or podcasts, begin your session at the start of a programme that doesn't last for longer than you are able to work for and stop when the programme ends. Followers of audiobooks can set a timer on their device so the book switches off after a chosen amount of time as their indication to take a break. Music lovers could create different length playlists for varying energy levels and select which one they work to. I find these techniques less reliable than using a timer as, whatever I'm listening to usually only exacerbates my urge for just a little bit more, but self-discipline may come more easily to you.

Instead of stopping

There are times when the complete rest that our body ultimately requires feels impossible. A need to distract yourself from pain, physiological restlessness in the body, or tiredness (let alone fatigue) resulting in poor impulse control, may be the culprits, but all is not lost – pacing doesn't always require that you grind to a complete halt. Sometimes the act of switching to another activity, or choosing the least strenuous distraction available to you, is enough to give your body an aspect of rest that is still helpful. Using different muscles, posture and cognitive skills allows the exercised parts of your body to take a break and recuperate. While this isn't a long-term strategy for those with energy-limiting conditions, it is better than continuing with one monotonous motion or thought process and can help you to wind down from your main activity.

Micro-resting, meanwhile, can be employed whatever you're doing and simply involves regularly taking 30 seconds to a minute or so of time out. Use this time to soften your gaze into the distance or close your eyes altogether, relax your muscles, exhale slowly and tune in to how your body is feeling before carrying on with what you were enjoying. As well as providing your body with moments of relaxation, developing this habit will enable you to become more aware of how your symptoms are responding to activity and whether continuing for much longer is advisable or not.

When pacing feels too hard

Whether in full crafting-flow or pursuing online entertainment, it takes self-awareness, discipline, patience and forethought to put down something you're enjoying because of a (possibly delayed) reaction brewing in your body.

When struggling with this, bear in mind Ovid's lesson from nature itself: 'Take rest; a field that has rested gives a bountiful crop.' Consider how happy you will be when you can pick up your tools again in a few hours or days because you chose to rest now. Remind yourself how cross, frustrated and disappointed you will feel if you forego pacing in favour of instant gratification, only to deplete your resources and be laid up in extended pain and stasis, wondering when, or even if, you'll return to your project. Give yourself reasons to trust in the strength of the long-term gain above and beyond momentary rewards and it becomes easier to find a sustainable pace that works for you.

Trust in the long-term gain above and beyond momentary rewards.

Sensible intentions and timers aren't always enough for me. (The irony that I ignored my timer while enthusiastically tapping out these words isn't lost on me.) However, I took a tip from parenting, downloaded a star chart app and assigned myself rewards for sticking to healthy limits. I thrive on achievements, so disappointment with a lack of stars on my chart provides me with a more immediate incentive than the nebulous prospect of delayed symptoms. It's not fool proof (as this fool can attest to) but has curbed my tendency to exceed what is sustainable for me, and rewarding myself with a treat when I reach a certain number of stars is always an added incentive!

There will be times when you go over your limit, either by mistake, or because you just really wanted to. It's not ideal but rarely is it irredeemable. We need to feel our way through our conflicting needs to find the balance that supports our long-term health while making the most of the moment at hand. Life isn't all about regimented rules, even if it feels that way when your body is being commandeered by a chronic health condition.

Sometimes spontaneity calls. When this happens, pace around the situation. Relinquish energy expenditure later that day, or the following day, in place of the activity you couldn't resist. Balance the over-exertion with an extended rest time or early night. Don't waste precious energy in berating yourself or worrying about the repercussions, but do take mitigating measures.

It's so easy to be cross that we can't indulge more time in our hobby, or to be resentful of our body's limitations, but this gets us nowhere other than bitterness and a tendency to push beyond our personal limits into increased symptoms. Instead, focus on the power held in those deliberate short periods of activity. When it comes to the frustration of having to cut back on what you enjoy, take a tip from gardening, where pruning a plant encourages more foliage and flowering in the long run.

Rather than being put off by the limitations your health places on your creative time, take heart that having to adhere to your body's requirements can at times become a tool as opposed to a hindrance. Psychologist Adam Alter points out that being constrained by a time limit frees us from extraneous thoughts, leaving our minds more able to focus. He suggests that this clarity is where great ideas are often born. So, when frustrated at having to down tools just as inspiration is flowing, jot down those sudden ideas, bank that enthusiasm for your next activity session, and remind yourself that having the freedom to work without limitations may have left you devoid of the stimulation to use it.

Rush neither to the finish line when the going is good, nor to defeat when brain fog or wobbly hands make so many wrong moves. Encourage yourself and give your body the space it needs to manoeuvre within the confines of its illness. If you must work more slowly than you'd like, consider how you could turn this into a positive. Slow stitching has become a trend, with books exalting the praises of this more meditative way of creating. Think of that – your sick body is trendy!

The value of something that has taken years to produce is immense. Some years ago, I wanted to knit myself a comfort blanket. I decided it would need to be constructed of many patches as I wouldn't be able to work with the weight of a whole blanket on my needles and, to keep myself motivated, I'd need the sense of fulfilment every time I completed a patch. I used chunky yarn and large needles to lower the workload, but it was still a big task. Sometimes I was only able to knit for minutes, sometimes closer to an hour. There were times when I would prop myself up in bed and risk ignoring, for a calculated period, my raised heart rate and laboured breathing, because I just wanted to have a go on it. At other times I didn't engage with it for weeks, maybe months, on end. It began to seem like a never-ending endeavour, but I carried on at the fluctuating pace my body dictated, overseen by self-care. One square at a time I worked on it, each completed block a mini achievement, and the pile of individual patches slowly grew. Three years later I completed my blanket, knitted not just with soft yarns but love and respect for myself and my needs, and this is what I wrap myself up in.

Taking time out

'My crafty meltdowns happen when I'm overtired,' a member of an online group once divulged to me. It can be difficult to admit that, just like an over-tired toddler, we need a nap or some time-out to get things back in perspective. Shouldn't we be in control of our emotional outbursts, riding out dipping energy levels with equilibrium and grace? Ha! Fatigue and persistent pain can make a toddler of the best of us, so let's embrace being tucked up with a snuggle blanket before overwhelm and tantrums take hold.

Resting, for us, may not be the enjoyable sensation that healthy people imagine it to be. We rest to the same old backdrop of pain and other distressing symptoms and not in welcome contrast to an active life. Reading for leisure, listening to music, watching TV, strolling in the countryside, soaking in a hot bath and all the other common suggestions for a restful break may be intensive activities for someone with severe chronic illness. My definition of resting involves lying flat with eyes shut, doing my best to ride out ever-present symptoms while wishing I could just get on with something interesting. Quite frankly, it can be hard and boring work.

> *When fizzy fidgets threaten to derail my time-out, imagining the actions that I'm abstaining from can form a bridge between doing them and full-on resting.*

If your body can relax to gentle music or spoken word these can occupy the brain enough for it to loosen its grip on runaway thoughts and desires. Podcasts, or the rhythm of an audiobook read by a good narrator, are how I trick my body into a more restful state, often resulting in sleep. When the jitters and fizzy fidgets threaten to derail my time-out, imagining the actions that I'm abstaining from can form a bridge between doing them and full-on resting, giving my body and mind something meditative to settle on as they wind down.

'My busy-bee brain agitates like a demented cheer-leader when I "lie about" and cannot "do",' says Marion who has severe ME. However, she knows the value of resting, not just for her sick body but as an act of rebellion in a society that rewards constant activity, production and tail-chasing. She reminds herself that 'Being is enough! Rest is radical!'

When feeling forced into stillness, it can help to recognise how we may have internalised negative messages about lying around, relaxing and not-doing, and consider turning this perspective around. In the past I have comforted myself by reciting the famous quote (attributed to Napoleon, speculating about China): 'Let her sleep, for when she wakes, she will shake the world.'

If you find a negative mindset around resting is truly ingrained and the frustration is huge, it may help to see your rest times as invisible work. You are working at internal regeneration, actively building energy reserves. Your brain is mulling over what you have been playing with and using this quiet time to subconsciously construct your next steps forward. Your job for now, and it's an important one, is to get out of the way so your body can do its thing. Sometimes resting is not only the most sensible but also the most productive option.

Even though you crave the hours of engagement that others can indulge in, take time to appreciate the bite-size portion of involvement you've been able to experience. Gratitude enables you to re-live the pleasure long after you've had to stop. Later, when you have gathered enough energy to indulge your eagerness, and your ideas are teetering on the outermost nest-edge of your mind, you can set a timer, pick up your tools and let yourself fly like a safely tethered kite amongst fledgling inspirations.

Suggested therapeutic activity

A reward jar

It's all too easy to resent the boredom and frustration of having to pace but we can motivate ourselves by associating taking a break with immediate good feelings. So, what pleasant rewards can you offer yourself every time you slow down and pause for a rest? Write out any ideas you have on slips of paper and store these in a container of your choice. Every time you successfully pace yourself, reach in and retrieve one.

Here are some suggestions to get you started:
- Tokens to pile up until you have enough to buy yourself a special treat

- Sentences that stimulate lovely memories for you to dwell on as you rest
- Supportive quotes
- Kind and encouraging messages to yourself
- Hug vouchers to redeem with willing participants
- Kiss cards to redeem with loved ones
- Prompts to cuddle a pet or a comforting soft toy
- Off-the-hook notes that permit you to abandon a specific chore in favour of full relaxation
- Congratulatory stickers.

From pushing to pacing at a glance

- Pacing will enable you to do more in the long run.
- Choosing to pace lowers the risk of being at the mercy of a body forcing you to draw to a complete halt.
- At times, pushing through symptoms may feel appropriate. Careful pacing the rest of the time can build reserves to cope with this.
- Be patient with your progress when learning new crafts or plodding through large projects.
- Little and often is best for ill bodies and for anyone learning new skills.
- Everyone's pace is unique to them and fluctuates over time.
- Using a timer can help you remember to take breaks. Factor in wind-down time rather than expecting yourself to stop abruptly.
- A micro-rest is better than no rest at all.
- 'Switching' activities so that you use different muscles, or cognitive instead of physical energy (and vice versa), is a form of pacing.
- Embrace the concept of resting as positive and pro-active. It is neither lazy nor unproductive.

Chapter 15
Good practice

Creativity has a reputation for spontaneity, with the muse in guiding position, but this isn't always the case. Developing a regular practice for your creativity will help you respond more effectively when inspiration does arrive. One member of the chronic illness community, who lives with ankylosing spondylitis, notes that her motivation to complete a sewing project is diminished when fatigue prevents her from enthusiastically diving into it. To combat this, she gives herself the target of a regular 15 minutes of sewing each day. Even when exhausted, she finds this achievable and has created a manageable framework that accommodates both her body and her creative practice.

Your practice needn't be daily. In fact, expecting this of yourself may result in despondency when medical needs, symptom flares and household responsibilities scupper your enthusiastic plans. If a daily commitment feels unsustainable, think on a broader scale. Your practice could include quiet meditation time when you let creative ideas percolate without intrusion. Allocate time and energy to creativity a few times a week or month. Keep your hands and mind dipped briefly but reassuringly regularly into the creativity pot, without putting any pressure on yourself to achieve impractical goals.

Be prepared

How many times have you fancied some creative fun only to find instead that a menial job you meant to sort out the other day has suddenly become urgent? Energy is diverted to this practicality and there goes another day passed without engaging your creative self. Instead, complete necessary life-tasks ahead of time whenever you can, timetabling extended rest and recuperation between activities. Prepare for the inevitability of unexpected chores or your illness taking the driving seat, rather than living with your energy so close to empty that you are completely halted by the unpredictability of life.

On planning your energy expenditure, actively apportion some time to creative fun. Telling yourself you will get stuck in when other necessities have been completed is another way of saying that your creativity isn't important to you. Build it into your timetable just as you would any other priority, not to pressure yourself into achieving anything but as a commitment to reserving energy for what you enjoy.

> *Build creativity into your timetable just as you would any other priority.*

Take time, also, to prepare for any upcoming medical appointments where you are likely to want a portable project you can whip out in a waiting room to occupy yourself with. Remember that you will be easily distracted by your surroundings and will have to stop work when summoned, so choose a project that doesn't require too much careful attention and can be abandoned and re-engaged with, with ease. If your area of interest isn't generally portable, consider what you might enjoy as an offshoot of your main craft. Machine sewers might like to dabble in English paper-piecing patchwork, where small shapes are sewn together by hand. Paper crafters who usually enjoy the precision of cutting their designs with a knife on a board may want to attend appointments with a small pack of origami paper for when bored or nervously needing to occupy their hands.

When feeling particularly unwell but not so ill that all crafting is out of the question, you will require something simple to distract yourself with. You might feel sure that, with the right materials on your lap, you could achieve something but reduced cognition and a body that feels like it's moving in quicksand simply isn't conducive to generating ideas or hunting out materials. Plan for this eventuality by preparing easy projects when in better phases so that you always have something ready to pick up when very simple occupational therapy is called for.

Having different projects on the go, each with varying cognitive and physical requirements, is a trick many artists use to help them through times of artistic ennui or creative blocks. For those of us with chronic conditions whose abilities fluctuate throughout one day, let alone a whole craft project, this practice has added benefits. If your muscles, like mine, struggle with repetitive actions, alternating different creative pursuits so that you vary which muscles, movements or sitting positions are used can extend your window of activity.

This is still applicable if you have just the one craft that you work with. Selina's ME and Meniere's disease allow her to knit regularly as long as she varies her hand movements, concentration levels and the way she holds her needles. To this end she ensures that she always has a selection of knitting projects prepared and to hand at any given moment, each of them calling for different sized needles, yarns or knitting techniques. While you may still have to limit your overall energy consumption, moving between activities in this way can eke out your abilities, preventing you from coming to such a rapid standstill or spending quite so long recovering.

Adapting to your needs

Sometimes we need to adapt either our expectations or practice to better suit our needs. When we consider this possibility, different crafts and aspects of life may become more available to us. Rather than persisting doggedly with a technique, style, piece of equipment, commitment or behaviour that is no longer supporting you and your body, alter the status quo. There is no reason why you should use tools or materials in the same way others do, or complete projects within an arbitrary time scale. Never fear that 'real' artists do it a certain way. On the contrary – this is how a creative mind makes the most of the situation it finds itself in. Adaptation, after all, guides evolution.

If your first choice of activity is beyond your body's abilities, then consider what your second choice would be or how your top preference could be adapted to something more manageable. How could you achieve the sensation or objective through a medium that lends itself more to your capabilities? Can't paint for various reasons? Perhaps you find you can 'paint' images with stitched threads or carefully chosen words, or collaged paper instead? If you love the feel of working with a paintbrush, perhaps you can embrace a more fluid style that doesn't require precise manual dexterity or detailed design?

Size matters

It is good practice throughout our creativity to consider how size can influence the effects of our chosen craft on our body and how achievable we find our goals. From the thickness of knitting needles, crochet hooks, paint brushes and pencils (or the use of grip aids to adjust these) to the size of our finished pieces, size is important.

Our goal is pleasure in our craft, and pleasure is harder to come by if our project causes so much discomfort that it begins to feel like a Sisyphean challenge.

Take patchwork and machine sewing, for example. Leaning across swathes of fabric to cut the required sizes, trying on clothes for fit as you make them, or holding the weight of a king-size patchwork quilt as you work on it may put your chosen craft beyond your means. Instead, I have often found patchwork motif greetings cards and cushion covers to be more accessible projects. If a quilt is your heart's dream, then a small lap quilt instead of one for the whole bed may be more achievable (and particularly useful for wheelchair users).

Knitters and crocheters who struggle with the stamina or strength involved in creating adult-sized clothing or blankets may find it easier to make hats, scarves, baby clothes or cot blankets to donate to charities and neonatal wards.

Think about how you can accommodate projects to suit you rather than compromising your needs to suit the project.

Chapter 15

Lara is a trained choreographer and dancer. When long-term illness landed on her body, she found herself exploring 'how to be a dancer with a body that can't often tolerate movement'. This resulted in her sharing a video online of a seamlessly edited montage of miniature dance sequences. Each section is only seconds long, featuring her wearing different clothes on new days in various spaces around her home. The effect could have been disjointed but the unifying factor holding it all together is her use of one song playing throughout. The result is captivating, communicating more than just the dance moves. By experimenting with how to adapt her expectations and allowing her body its limitations, Lara found a method for expressing her art in illness-friendly portions from which she could later build a full-length piece.

> *How can you accommodate projects to suit you rather than compromising your needs to suit the project?*

We can exploit Lara's technique in other areas of creativity that size has made forbidding, breaking them down into tiny portions, perhaps presenting these as they arrive in miniature or patching them together.

Perhaps, for now, an idea for a novel could be experimented with as micro-fiction, or a series of short stories that build into a more epic tale, or exploration on a theme. Embarking on each piece individually, without the complex planning of a full novel could give a neglected idea the chance to exist in some form. Practise diversifying in this way to embrace what your body is capable of. Poetry, especially haiku, flash fiction, brief prose vignettes and stickperson-illustrated graphic stories are all ways of channelling literary ideas into bite-size pieces that those with limited physical resources may feel better able to achieve.

Scaling down could reveal a newfound passion. Have you always loved the idea of topiary but ladders, hedge cutters and unstable limbs just don't mix? How about tending and shaping a bonsai tree or dwarf shrub instead? Find as many hacks as you can to adjust to what is hindering you.

Of course, smaller isn't always quicker or easier. I have lamented to novel writers that I can only manage very short stories, to be met with their admiration for my genre. They find novels an easier task than making each word powerfully justify its space in a condensed form. Similarly, tight stitches, detailed work, and fine accuracy can sometimes take more of a toll on us than loosely generous, baggy or large brushstroke creations. Imagine your passion is beading but your fine motor skills, muscle-shakes or limited vision preclude you from this fiddly craft. Perhaps sizing up would be an option rather than having to abandon what you enjoy? Larger beads could create wall decorations, hanging baskets or other unusual statement pieces.

Whether you scale up or scale down, let your body lead the way into creations that work for you. The unique techniques instigated by your health may even make a trendsetter of you.

Know your shortcuts from your dead ends

Don't be tempted to cut corners because of fatigue, pain or limited time. Take it from one who has done this and knows: you will likely regret it! By all means, adapt and experiment with different tricks and tools, but some laborious techniques or preparations are worth adhering to. They may appear to slow you down but will save you from having to rectify problems later.

Too often I have felt too tired to protect my clothes from paint that may want to escape, or have relied on scanty pinning rather than preliminary tacking, only to spend far more energy backing out of these dead-end actions than if I'd taken a bit more care in the first place. Scrimping on the preparatory stages, or ignoring your instinct that something isn't right, is a false energy economy.

Always measure at least twice before cutting, double-check instructions, protect your surroundings from messy equipment, put in place any safety measures (including supportive cushions), do your research, and fetch your timer if it's in another room.

Work as well as you can, not as fast as you can. Uncertainty as to when we'll next be well enough to make progress can tempt us into getting as much done as possible right now. Wisdom, however, reminds us that less haste often results in greater speed. Be prepared to give proper attention to the process of your craft, so as to get the most out of yourself and your materials. It will be worth it in the long run. Your energy is precious but so are your creations, so make it your practice to give them their due care.

Playing as practice

Remember that the point of your creativity is to enjoy something your body can do and to build feel-good vibes within. We may say that we're 'working' on a project but to describe it as play could be just as accurate and lift any self-imposed pressure that might undermine our desire to reduce stresses on our body and mind.

Give a project space to grow organically, playing with whatever is at your disposal. My best textile creativity emerges not from any clear vision but when playing with scraps of fabric and moving colours around in front of me. Whether due to brain fog or simply the way my mind functions, I rarely develop a clear image of an outcome until my playthings have guided me. While a larger project gradually develops, or when symptoms insist I put it on the back burner, I toy with other creative outlets and concepts. These often surprise me by becoming more satisfying than the 'proper work' I have had to step away from.

Keep your engagement with creativity alive, even when you don't feel up to a full-blown project, by laying out various materials and moving them around with no other intent than to enjoy their colours, textures and combinations. Photograph anything pleasing that emerges before moving it all apart and starting again. Later, after a regathering of energy, you might use your photographs as a launch-pad for a more permanent creation. Jot down words in fun combinations without any intention of producing something coherent. Play with the feel of your favourite pen or instrument in your hands.

Have fun exploring your expectations of your work and your chosen routes to results. Through a playful attitude, challenge your responses to the world and how both your body and materials can be used.

Challenge your responses to the world and how both your body and materials can be used.

Look at the wrong side of textiles, photos turned upside down, words in an unusual order, objects in unexpected roles, your weaknesses highlighted to advantage.

Experiment playfully with perceptions. Your body doesn't operate according to the standard user's manual and neither need your creativity. Be free with your fun and let your creative play become what it will – a grand masterpiece, a grand disaster or anything in between.

Spread your wings, then assess the view

Some people find one creative airstream that they settle into and, for them, this works well. I, however, have found it good practice to spread my creative wings and dip into different currents. The disappointment when my body hasn't been able to maintain my chosen path, or when a project hasn't panned out as intended, is ameliorated by having another area of creativity to turn to. A variety of skills is both stimulating and allows you to remain adaptable, depending on your body's changing needs.

In the past, I would disparage my butterfly approach to crafting, calling myself a Jack-of-all-trades in comparison to those who focused on excelling in one area. Then I learnt that while we now use the curtailed sentence derogatively, the original adage affirmed that 'A Jack of all trades is master of none, but is often times better than a master of one.' It certainly puts me at an advantage when having to vary muscular movements and cognitive abilities. The cartoonist Gilbert Sullivan recognises how his career has been enhanced by being reasonably good at a few disciplines (business, drawing and jokes) rather than brilliant at just one. Moving between different skill-sets unlocks

Chapter 15

innovation, both at a design level and in cross-referencing practical solutions to physical difficulties.

Every so often, just as you must assess whether your body requires a change of posture, different movements, a short break or total rest, take a moment to assess the overview of your craft path. Is it bringing you pleasure and gentle stimulation? If not, is it serving you in some other way that is worth the energy you are expending on it? What would you really like to be doing right now, regardless of whether it aligns with your preconceptions about your skill-set? If you have the urge to tilt your wings in a new direction, then investigate how this could be possible for you.

When it comes to assessing individual creative pieces, I have realised that my responses share much with my body's response to energy usage. Just as I need extended time for delayed symptomatic reactions to fully emerge and then subside, I now know also to give my varied responses to my creations time to come to the fore and settle.

Neither post-activity-exhaustion nor the adrenaline high precipitated by my body trying to rise above pain or fatigue are conducive to clarity of thought, however much I believe otherwise in the moment. If, at a project's completion, I'm buoyed up on the buzz of success I will likely later fall into realisation of the faults and alterations to be addressed. Conversely, if I finish a piece feeling dejected it usually just needs setting aside for a while before I realise there's a lot (or at least something) in its favour. Giving yourself space to arrive at a more objective assessment of your work may save you from rash decisions or physically draining emotions.

If, after time, you still doubt your constructive critical faculties, I recommend looking at visual art in a mirror, or listening to recordings of yourself playing your instrument or reading your writing aloud. Second opinions are great but not always easy to come by when unable to attend groups or discuss your work with other interested parties. By seeing your work reflected in reverse, or hearing it at one remove via a recording, your powers of objectivity are placed in a stronger position to assess your work for yourself.

Suggested creative exercise
A commitment certificate

Think realistically about the minimum amount of time you could regularly and enjoyably (absolutely no self-pressure allowed!) engage in arts or crafts. Are there any less measurable ways you intend to develop your creativity, too? Write these all down in the form of vows to your creative self. Now, make a certificate declaring your commitment. You can make it as official looking or wildly decorative as you desire. Keep it somewhere to hand, as a reminder of your intentions to establish a regular practice and generally expand your creative outlook.

Good practice at a glance

- Fostering a regular practice can provide motivation when illness or daily life is dragging your enthusiasm down.
- To prevent avoidable discouragement, make your regular practice as achievable as possible (considering the fluctuations of life and illness). This could be five minutes a day, half an hour a month – whatever feels sustainable to you.
- Adapt to your body's specific needs and qualities.
- Have projects of different sizes and skills on the go, to suit varying moods and functional capacity.
- Be wary of taking shortcuts in your creative projects that may lead to problems in the long run.
- Play and experimentation are forms of creative practice.
- Observe your work and your body objectively in order to make wise decisions.

Chapter 16
Recovering from perfectionism

If you're hesitating from exploring creative pursuits because your health prevents you from proficiency in your desired craft, or a perceived lack of talent renders anything you create unworthy of your respect, this may well be perfectionism tricking you. Because here's the thing: perfection is not a prerequisite for creativity. More to the point, it is not conducive to a creative life. It can help with the finishing touches (if it ever lets you finish) but not the all-important ability to get started and simply enjoy being creative. Therefore, the tendency towards perfectionism or self-criticism is an important topic if we are having difficulty comforting ourselves with our own creativity.

Illness and its toxic partner, perfectionism

Chronic illness affects all personality types from all walks of life. However, those with strong ambition and firm goals may be more likely to impose stress on their body by pushing through symptoms until their body declares, with scant room for negotiation, that it has had enough. Some of us held in the grip of tricky symptoms may have this long-held leaning towards high attainment.

For others, the illness itself might trigger this perfection-seeking mind-set. If meticulous planning and accessibility don't run smoothly, our lives are not just inconvenienced, they grind to a halt. Trapped in a body that doesn't respond to even the fiercest will, there is an urge to gain control over other aspects of life and to prove one's ability to actualise desires. In addition, those of us with dynamic disabilities (that is, a disability with fluctuating symptoms and severity), influenced by all kinds of variables, are often plagued by the sense that we must live with perfect vigilance at all times. We only have to take our eye off our behavioural strategies momentarily and weeks' worth of progress or carefully maintained stability can come tumbling down. Perfectionism tricks us into thinking it holds the answer when, in fact, our condition is inconsistent, and the unpredictability of life needs living.

Like any toxic partner, perfectionism isn't all bad. After all, there must be something about it that attracted us to it in the first place. At its most helpful, a desire for perfection urges us to commit to doing our best and working on what we know we can improve. In excess, however, it pushes us further than is healthy. It triggers stress responses at the physical level while eating away at self-confidence. At its cruellest, it convinces us that nothing we make is worthy of our time, money or energy, let alone other people's attention. It tells us not to embarrass ourself with substandard attempts. 'It's just protecting me from disappointment,' you might justify. Well, yes, you may be protected from certain disappointments but this is primarily perfectionism's disappointment, and it keeps you from the fun of any involvement at all.

Trapped in a body that doesn't respond to even the fiercest will, perfectionism tricks us into thinking it holds the answer.

Alternative A's

We have enough battles to attend to when living with chronic illness without inventing more. So, are you feeling ready to drop that 'A-star' mindset that demands outstanding achievement and perceived perfection? If so, let's turn our attention towards two alternative A's:

Accommodate your shortcomings and any difficulties you encounter due to your health. Let them into your creative space and work with them. Remember that they may even enhance the individuality of what you produce. For example, I know that I am not good at precise work. I am also often so limited in energy that I require shortcuts when assembling textile and paper art, so I have adopted the practice of fraying fabric edges and tearing paper.

It's a trick to hide my difficulties that has become a signature feature. I have learnt to circumnavigate a limitation and, in doing so, found a personal style. Accommodation of your imperfections and illness, rather than making your work inferior, may be the origin of your speciality. Accommodating an unchosen element takes courage and hope, both of which are virtues to be proud of, whatever the outcome.

Accept that it might take you a while to find where you best fit and to reach a standard that you can be happy with. Even then, it may take you longer to bring your creations into existence than other people seem to require, with extended periods of time when you are too ill to work on anything, but your creativity can hibernate without being presumed missing. Accept that if you choose to push yourself into new areas of expertise some of your attempts will be disasters. It is okay to dislike aspects of your work without feeling the need to write it off as a failure or doubt your validity as a creator. Creativity isn't all or nothing, and difference is not the same as 'better than' or 'worse than'. There are some things you will never be brilliant at or able to engage in and this is okay. Indeed, it may be more than okay. It is imperfection that makes every one of us relatable. What we are really learning to do here, is to accept ourselves. Living in a society that is so often afraid or ignorant of chronic illness, many of us have internalised the message that being something other than our imperfect, ill or disabled selves is what we should be striving for and, if that isn't possible, to be as unobtrusive as possible. How about we accept that our challenge, in life and creativity, is to be more of ourselves, regardless of any perfection myths?

Starting with confusion and mess

Sometimes just starting makes the unimaginable achievable, so give something – anything – a go. Jabeen is a chronically ill painter who advises, 'Make something imperfect for no reason and no need to prove anything.' Just like navigating a chronic illness, the process of creativity often lends itself to feeling like you have no idea what you're doing. Give yourself space to be utterly inept and see what comes from experimentation. Simply beginning to bring an idea into the physical world is an achievement, regardless of its aesthetic quality. You may make an almighty mess, but this is often the route in. You may even end up loving the mess.

Take this book. Somewhere between jotting down initial thoughts and typing coherent sentences I lost faith. I had no more ideas. How was I even well enough to pull together a unified book-length manuscript? Refusing to give in to self-doubt, I wrote without censorship. I scribbled disjointed thoughts, recorded random memories. My jumbled notes were so far from perfect that much of it was unusable, but I kept on. Little by little, curiosity and determination led the way. Over time, the concept morphed. I played with paragraphs like the pieces of a jigsaw puzzle without a picture on the box. I scrapped a lot but it was neither a sign of inadequacy nor wasted energy. My thoroughly imperfect musings, trials and errors were invaluable in leading me here.

Perfectionism does not realise that some of the best conclusions come from accidents and diverted paths. It cannot see that imperfections can have an appeal of their own. We could consider diamonds and the imperfections in them being what reflect the light so stunningly. Speaking of diamonds, Virginia Woolf referred to her diary as a dustheap from which she could extract literary diamonds, which just goes to show that even the outpourings of lauded artists don't spill from them perfectly formed and may never develop into anything they would choose to share.

Some of the best conclusions come from accidents and diverted paths.

While every creator has their own limitations, as carriers of chronic illness, our own are somewhat heavier than we'd often like to admit. We can forget what is caused by the devastation of illness and, instead, criticise ourselves for less-than-ideal practice and outcomes. Just as you crave gentle treatment and compassionate care when you navigate a life governed by ill health, transfer that feeling to your creativity. Hold it carefully and offer encouragement when it flails. Find something of value in the mess. For creative ideas to be safe to explore beyond the confines of your mind they require the freedom to be imperfect. They need to be allowed to trip up, fall down, look silly and develop in their own way. Embrace the vast disasters and miniature successes. And when doubting the value of your latest mess, consider whether its current state is just a stage it's going through. With time and more attention, perhaps it will grow out of its ugly phase.

Not that 'getting better' need be your objective. I am no more proficient at piano playing than I was as a teenager, certainly in part because of my reduced capacity for practice. I have come to accept this and enjoy making the music that I can. My knitting and writing skills, however, have expanded. I pick and choose my creative avenues according to my current health situation and whatever I feel connected to. I am learning that what happens next is part of the adventure rather than a hallowed destination.

So, instead of setting your sights on perfect results, start with where you are and see where that may take you. Dip your toes in. Mess around. Fiddle with materials, doodle, free-associate, and play with minor risks. Celebrate and integrate the unexpected, the divergent and the atypical in yourself and your creations. Set realistic goals and hold on to the conviction that you are determined enough to reach whatever potential is available to you. In time, you will feel bolder as you see themes and strengths emerge.

Continuing to make mistakes

It has been said that the difference between a master and a beginner is that the master has failed more times than the beginner has tried. It is so easy to linger on our mistakes, uneven tension, imbalanced compositions and human imperfections but, given time and a healthier perspective, they can take on a different import. Knowing what *will* work is often presaged by having discovered what does *not* work. I was taught to always re-draw the mark I had intended to make before erasing the first faulty one. My errors are valuable guides to where *not* to put my pencil. So, stay open to the errors as much as the triumphs.

Selina, a knitter who suffers with ME and Meniere's disease, started learning to knit as something to do when sitting at home day after day. She doesn't unduly fret about her errors, saying that 'In Tanzania it is regarded as bad luck if a creation is perfect and so the craftsperson always makes a deliberate mistake. This is why I accept mistakes and tend to leave them, because they reflect life which is never perfect.' When energy is drastically limited, making mistakes can feel like a devastating waste of your rationed supply so becoming more sanguine about leaving some errors in your work is one way of conserving energy. But what about when your error can't be saved? Or when not saving is the mistake itself?

During a particularly brain-foggy phase of writing this book I forgot to regularly save what I was typing, repeatedly making the additional mistake of selecting the 'Don't Save' option when closing my document. I was devastated at what I perceived as a pointless waste of time and energy, but Lior, an online friend, had wise words to share: 'I think the practice of writing, even if you don't keep hold of the results, is valuable in itself. You got the satisfaction of having written and having been able to use your brain.' She was right. Casting our attention in a creative direction, when illness threatens to consume us, is a constructive act in itself.

Allow space for trial, error and daft mistakes within your work and management of your health. You might find that the mishaps and aborted ideas become as valuable as the successes.

The following poem is the result of accepting and integrating a fundamental mistake I had made in its concept. Halfway through drafting the poem in my mind I realised I had miscalculated how long I had been unwell for and came to the temporary conclusion that this made the whole premise of the poem defunct – until it occurred to me that incorporating this error into the poem could be the solution. To my joy, this led to greater poignancy and originality than my initial idea had envisioned.

Eternity

> I spoke to myself
>   About writing a poem called
>   Thirty-three point three recurring
> It would connect my
>   Thirty-three years of illness
>   With the mathematical
> Phenomenon of
>   Repetition into
>   Infinity, only
> I wasn't sure I
>   Could handle the metaphor,
>   Maths not being my---
> I don't like to interrupt,
>   I whispered, but actually
>   It's thirty-seven
> At least thirty-seven
>   Years with this illness.
>   Maybe more.

Even those mistakes that you feel have taught you nothing may yet become stepping stones. They have instructed you in something, if only in what not to do next time or to be more gentle with yourself in the face of failure. How about cataloguing your so-called failures as an *Anthology of Accidents*? When reviewing them, enjoy recognising how far you've come, look for qualities you can work with, and know that these previous disappointments have helped create the ever-developing you.

Choosing satisfaction

What is it that you find most satisfying about creating: the process or the product? When this question was asked in an online creativity group for those with chronic illness, the majority responded that they were in it for the process. If that is the case for you, don't get overly hung up on the quality of your finished piece. 'Creating for the sake of it,' observes Andy who has lived with ME for over two and half decades, 'we can infuse everything we touch with both the joy of creation and pain of whatever we are going through. Do we create masterpieces? Rarely, but each moment of joy can be its own masterpiece.'

Embrace the satisfaction of simply partaking in your chosen activity at whatever level you can. For some, it is the rhythm of the movement that appeals to them. Others are drawn to an activity that lets the mind wander freely. Some appreciate freedom of expression. None of these enjoyments is focused on the outcome of the piece or how long it takes to get there. This is something I have struggled with. However, by practising letting go of so much emphasis on the final product, I am making progress. I am learning to enjoy the journey rather than always looking ahead for the desired destination.

'Do we create masterpieces? Rarely, but each moment of joy can be its own masterpiece.' – Andy

When things don't go to plan, I try to examine the situation with curiosity rather than concerning myself with whether my work will impress others or not. Virginia Woolf journaled about this, saying that writing delighted her when she engaged in it for the pure love of the act rather than caring what others thought.

Not bothering what anyone says includes sometimes ignoring your own inner critic. When the temptation to bemoan how the quality, speed or style of your work differs from your desires, consider the observation made by art historian Luis-Martin Lozano regarding one of Frida Kahlo's less well-known artworks, painted at the end of her life. He noted that although her body and brain were not able to portray exactly what she wanted, the imperfect result was still a powerful painting that deserved to be seen.

Perfection be damned. You are doing the best you can, so give yourself credit for everything you do achieve under the weight of chronic illness.

Good enough is good enough.

Suggested creative exercise
Embracing imperfection

This activity is inspired by my experience with Lisa Congdon's Daily Drawing Challenge on Creativebug. You will need a page of plain paper, a pen (not a pencil or anything erasable, and preferably not a biro – you'll get more satisfying results from a fine fibre tip pen), and a prompt from the box below. Whichever prompt you choose, draw as many different representations of it as you like. These can be realistic, impressionistic or stylistic. You can draw from imagination, from images online, or from objects around you. The only rule is that you erase or reject nothing. Be brave and keep going even when you make a 'wrong' mark. Work with it, develop it, incorporate it, build upon it, or just let it be.

You may want to choose one prompt a day/week and see how you develop. Your abilities will probably lend themselves to some styles and techniques better than others. It is ok to not be good at them all. Hopefully, as you practice this activity, your comfort levels around imperfect results will strengthen.

Trees Fish Cakes Leaves Suns Eyes Footwear Nests

Spoons Daisies Hats Stars Feathers Arrows Teapots

Webs Keys Kites Bottles Spirals Boats

Recovering from perfectionism at a glance

- A desire for the perfect end result can stop us from even starting.
- Creativity is not dependent on ideal outcomes.
- Chronic illness can exacerbate a need to control how things turn out.
- Accommodate your creative imperfections so that you integrate them into your work.
- Accept that it may take time to master a craft and that you will experience failed attempts.
- Embrace messy and confused efforts. You never know where they may take you.
- It is okay to make mistakes. Every mistake has something to teach us.
- Our mistakes may even lead to original work.
- Even artists with great skill will never feel satisfied when chasing perfection.
- We can choose when to be satisfied with our work.
- Satisfaction can come from enjoying how we pass our time and not the end product.

Chapter 17
Create-ability

Not every craft or art technique we'd like to involve ourselves in will be possible, but some abstract problem-solving and research into adaptations can open our doorway into the craft world a little wider. Some of the tips and equipment mentioned in this chapter will be familiar to seasoned artists and crafters, but those of us with disabling illness may find ourselves needing them for even very short creativity sessions, either to enable the activity in the first place or to prevent further pain and fatigue from developing.

After nearly four decades of crafting with chronic illness I am still discovering ways to make creativity more accessible. The trick is to use whatever help is available before you think you really need it. It is easier to take precautionary measures than it is to wait for your body to recover from increased pain and fatigue.

Student without a class

Learning from books alone, when not well enough to attend a class or group, does put us chronically ill at a disadvantage. It's true that there's no substitute for someone with experience demonstrating what we're not grasping from diagrams and written instructions. This is where technology becomes our saviour.

YouTube tutorials are fabulous for bringing an expert into our room. There's no embarrassment about asking for repeated demonstrations when we can pause and replay the lesson as often as needed. By choosing the option to watch the tutorial at a slower playback speed you can really scrutinise the manoeuvres and get a grip on what's required. I gave up on my attempts at learning crochet from a library book but watching online lessons enabled me to master some basic crochet projects.

If a relative, friend or fellow member of an online group has a skill that you're struggling with, consider connecting with them via video-call. They will be able to spot where you may be going wrong and guide you in the right direction. My first foray into macramé was achieved this way. I have also made very short videos (just a couple of minutes long) on my phone, teaching friends basic textile techniques far more successfully, and using less energy, than if I tried to type out the explanation or explain it over the phone without a visual demonstration.

Memory aids

Fatigue, cognitive impairment and brain fog can all hamper our ability to learn new skills. One way of helping yourself through this is to talk out loud to yourself. As well as reading or watching instructions, listen to your voice verbalising them. This uses your attention more holistically, with different parts of your brain working together to process and retain the information. Speaking to yourself in the second person, using your name as you speak encouragingly to yourself, helps cement the instructions and increase self-control, reducing the risk of becoming cross with yourself or giving up in frustration.

Until actions become habitual, memory issues can be particularly problematic. Reciting the order of repetitive actions as rhymes or short narratives – e.g., 'In, and around, and through, and off' for the actions that create a basic continental knit stitch – is an age-old technique. A macabre modern recitation for the common English knit stitch goes: 'stab him' (as you poke the right-hand needle into the stitch on your left-hand needle), 'strangle him' (wrap the yarn around the right-hand needle), 'scoop out his guts' (bring this

Using your name as you speak encouragingly to yourself helps cement the instructions and increase self-control.

needle back through the working stitch, carrying the wrapped yarn with it), 'push him off the cliff' (push the stitch that you were working with off the end of the left-hand needle). 'In through the front door, go round the back, out through the window, jump off Jack' is a more traditional rhyme for the same stitch. Meanwhile, 'In through the back way, then rope the hog, back out the gate, and jump off the log' guides the learner knitter through the movements that make up purl stitch. Those new to macramé sometimes recite the rhyme 'Right over left, left over right, makes a knot both tidy and tight' to help them into the rhythm of the commonly used square (or reef) knot.

Mnemonics for sequences are also incredibly helpful. Three and a half decades of piano playing and I can still sometimes be heard muttering '**G**reat **B**ig **D**iamonds **F**rom **A**frica' and '**A**ll **C**ows **E**at **G**rass' to remind myself of the musical notes on the lines and spaces of the bass clef. The adage '**E**very **G**ood **B**oy **D**eserves **F**ootball' and the acronym FACE are the most popular aides memoire for the treble clef.

Creating your own mnemonic that you can recite to the tune of a familiar song or nursery rhyme is one way of making any information stick more securely in your mind.

From shoulder to finger

Shaky hands are a real encumbrance to any craft that requires fine motor skills. My shakes are caused by weak muscles, so supporting my arms and hands on a cushion, tray or table is helpful in reducing this symptom. Neurologists sometimes suggest weighted cuffs on the wrists to ease arm tremors, especially those associated with Parkinson's disease. A Helping Hand or Third Hand tool that either stands on or clamps to a surface and holds items aloft for you is great when more than two hands are required but also helpful if your own hands can't hold something steady enough to work with precision.

Many types of grip aid are available for people with limited strength or grip ability. These can be attached to a variety of standard, narrow tools such as crochet hooks, pens, pencils and paint brushes to enable better dexterity and less pain. Abiligrip is popular, while Functionalhand holds items at a more comfortable angle for some.

Finger splints and yokes are helpful for those who have pain or difficulty moving digits due to arthritis or loose ligaments. They support the joints, helping prevent both partial and full dislocations as well as overextension. Metal splints are considered more effective by some crafters than the plastic ones provided by the NHS. Many choose ring splints that allow for a range of movement and look less medical, some designed to resemble fashionable rings.

Pain in the shoulders, hands, wrists and digits that is caused by repetitive strain may benefit from the use of wrist splints or compression gloves that support the muscles and tendons. These come in the form of complete gloves, wrist supports and thumb supports as well as neoprene wrist, shoulder and upper arm braces. Although not a cure that will allow me to ignore my symptoms, I have found the wrist and thumb support gloves comfortable and supportive when knitting, typing, writing or piano playing.

Many crafts involve cutting something at some point or another, but sore joints, weak muscles and sensitivity to pressure can make using scissors at best uncomfortable and at worst impossible. There are alternatives to standard scissors, from electric, easy-grip or spring action (also known as self-opening) to rotary cutters, 360° rotating cutting tools, one finger cutters, and more. Once you know these options exist it's worth investigating what could suit you better than the traditional scissors you may have been doggedly persevering with.

Holding books open when reading for research or following patterns and recipes has been made infinitely easier for me by a Book Seat. This is a specially shaped beanbag that sits on your lap or the bed with a ledge for your book to rest on and a low Perspex strip that holds the pages open. Book couches serve a similar purpose, while Book Chairs and traditional cookery book stands are best used only on smooth, flat surfaces. If holding the book isn't a problem but you need help keeping the pages open, a Book Thumb or a Gimble are both options.

Reaching and reclining

Reaching for dropped items, or having to get up and down from your chosen place, uses valuable energy that could be better spent on what you enjoy and is no fun when you've finally found a position resembling comfort, so keep an easily accessible toolbox, basket or bag within reach that contains everything you're likely to need throughout your craft session. Wheelchair side bags with compartments can be bought that hang from the outside of the arm of the chair. A bespoke storage system would make a great craft project in itself. A grabber reaching-stick to retrieve fallen items could prove useful, too.

Not being able to sit up at a table to craft can pose problems but these are usually resolvable with some research to find what adaptive surface most suits you. Over-bed tilt tables and laptop stands that either swivel or wheel away when not in use are invaluable to some. I love my bed tray that hides under the bed until I retrieve it. It has an adjustable top that can be tilted to a selection of angles, making it more ergonomic for drawing or typing, and legs that fold out to hold it over my lap rather than imposing any weight on me. Some have split tops so you can angle the portion that you're painting on while keeping the remainder flat for pots of water or ink. Lap trays on a beanbag base that settle to the shape of you are a good option if you can tolerate weight on your legs.

If you find yourself working from a wheelchair, specifically shaped wheelchair lap trays are available to save you from balancing things precariously on your lap. Meanwhile, adjustable desktop drawing boards may be a solution for those who like to use an easel but don't find their mobility enables this.

If you're able to sit upright and unsupported and find yourself working at varying heights of work surface, or on a dressmaker's dummy, then a stool is worth investing in. Bar stools and perch seats are great for working at countertop height, but if you need to be slightly higher so that you are raised enough for your shoulders to be comfortably dropped (when mixing things in a bowl on a kitchen surface, for example) then I wholly recommend an artist's stool or draughtsman's chair. The seat of an artist's stool is attached to a large central screw that can be swivelled around to adjust the sitting height, while a draughtsman's chair has a lever action to adjust the seat height and the addition of wheels, enabling you to scoot around your room.

Knitting and crochet

Whether knitting or crocheting, if you are experiencing pain in your hands or arms, experiment with different size hooks and needles. Larger ones (referring to their diameter, rather than length) are usually easier to hold with a looser grip, thus reducing the likelihood of pain.

In both crochet and knitting, the larger the needles or hook the bigger the stitches. Used in conjunction with chunkier yarn, or two or more strands of DK yarn at once, you will be able to create items much more quickly than when using smaller gauge needles and yarn. Some people find they struggle just as much with very thick needles and hooks as they do with delicate ones and that there is a sweet spot in the middle that is most comfortable for them. Mine is aran weight, chunky or two strands of DK yarn on 4-6 mm needles. With a little experimentation you will find which size range brings you the most ease.

If you are a knitter who finds the weight of chunky yarn puts too much of a strain on your wrists as your knitting grows, a compromise that works for some is lace knitting. This is very delicate and airy, using lightweight yarn on 4 mm needles.

Chapter 17

When following a pattern that requires a smaller crochet hook than you are comfortable holding, ergonomic hooks will be worth investigating. These have chunky, easier to grip, ergonomically shaped handles that don't affect the size of the working end of the hook. Alternatively, you can make an existing crochet hook easier to hold in the palm of your hand by wedging an egg-shaped makeup sponge along the length of the crochet hook.

An ergonomic style of knitting needle is the square needle, so called because were you to cut a cross section of it you would see a square rather than round shape. While these may sound strangely uncomfortable to hold, they are said to be easier to grip than traditional needles and gentler on the joints.

Bear in mind that the material of your needles can play a part in how easily you manoeuvre them and how their temperature affects your joints. I love my Nanna's cool-to-the-touch metal knitting needles that slide smoothly through the stitches, but bamboo and wooden needles have become very popular, especially for those with arthritis, for their light weight and natural warmth.

Bed- or sofa-bound knitters may find that supportive cushions and pillows hinder the movement of long needles. If your project doesn't require many stitches in each row, shorter needles – even children's ones – may be a simple answer. Many find circular needles easier to work with when having to remain lying down or semi-prone. These also have the advantage of spreading the weight of large projects more evenly across their length rather than pulling heavily on one needle and tiring your hand. Some people also place large projects in a bowl on their lap that they can easily spin when they need to turn their work.

Circular needles are easier to work with when having to remain lying down or semi-prone.

Whatever type of knitting needle you opt for, hold them as gently or loosely as possible, letting them rest in your back three fingers with the length of the needles wedged against your palm for extra leverage rather than relying solely on your fingers and thumbs. This allows you to manoeuvre just the tips of the needles with minimal hand movement. Keeping your arms close to you rather than stretched out in front or elbows stuck out to the side will help prevent shoulder-blade pain and numbness in hands.

An issue, other than grip, with smaller knitting needles is how sharp their point can be. This is important for ease of poking through small stitches but, after a while, results in sore fingertips, especially if your nerves are sensitive, and can even cause nerve damage. Silicone thimbles are a handy solution, as are rubber-ring fingertip grips (these have an open top so are perfect if you have long nails). They are flexible, fit well and incorporate breathing holes so your fingers don't sweat. Adjustable metal thimbles are also available, if you're more of a traditionalist, as well as leather thimbles.

I grew up assuming the way my Nanna taught me to knit was the only option, but different regions have their own methods. Investigating a variety of techniques will give you alternatives that may be easier on your body. Having the ability to alternate between different styles is a bonus when joints and muscles need a change of movement.

Portuguese knitting uses a pin attached to your shoulder to guide the yarn through. This can be helpful for visually impaired knitters as the yarn stays put and is easier to find. If you struggle with tangled yarns when knitting with different colours this technique will help with that, providing you thread each yarn through a different pin. According to Andrea Wong, who teaches Portuguese knitting, little movement is needed to form the stitches, making this a good alternative for people with carpal tunnel syndrome, arthritis, and joint pain. If you want to give it a go without buying extra accessories, you can loop the yarn around your neck instead of threading it through a pin. Alternatively, fashion a homemade Portuguese style knitting pin from a small binder clip attached to a safety pin or by hanging an earring hook upside down from a brooch or safety pin.

Chapter 17

Lever-action knitting, also known as Irish cottage or pivot knitting, and most like English knitting, has traditionally been used by production knitters because it allows for faster work with reduced risk of pain. It involves steadying one of the needles under your arm to reduce fatigue. Traditional Scottish knitters use extra-long (35-40 cm) needles similarly. Those of you who don't get on with circular needles and knit in the round with long double pointed needles (DPNs) may benefit from a traditional Shetland knitting belt. Also known as a makkin belt (makkin being the Shetland word for knitting), it is made from stuffed leather with holes on the front and worn on the right arm. The holes are there to hold the end of your DPNs, stabilising them for you, speeding up your work and helping maintain balanced tension while easing any wrist strain. The makkin belt is also sometimes used to help with lever-action knitting and has the added advantage of creating very even work.

I have had periods of time when one arm has been out of action while the other was useable. This is incredibly frustrating when you know you could enjoy an activity if only it didn't rely on both arms. Only recently did I discover that knitting can be carried out one-handedly. Traditionally, this was considered the norm in some areas to enable mothers and workers to knit while holding a baby or tending to other duties. Knitting sheaths, made of leather or wood, were attached to the knitter's belt around their waist or held under their arm and this held the static needle for them. A search online for one-handed knitting tutorials will result in videos and text tutorials to guide you through the process. Some suggest you hold the second needle clamped under your arm, others will tell you about aids that can be bought, such as the Knitting Aid that sits on your lap and holds one or both needles for you. One-handed crocheting is also possible and, again, there are online tutorials to guide you through this.

Anna, a keen knitter whose crafting is limited by living with ME, was pleased to discover that continental knitting proved easier on her hands and arms than the more traditional English knitting. Continental knitting uses the left, rather than the right hand to hold the working yarn and, for this reason, crocheters tend to find it easier to get along with when branching out into knitting.

Having found a method that better suits her hands, the symptom that now impedes Anna's knitting progress the most is brain fog. The complicated colour work that she is so good at requires concentration that is hard for her to maintain. Having a selection of row counters (one for each knitting project on the go) will help you keep track of exactly where in the pattern you are, even if you are forced to take considerable time away from your project. Basic analogue counters and more fancy electronic ones both work well. There are also apps, many of them free, to help knitters and crocheters note exactly which stitch as well as row they are working on.

Stitch markers are a common tool in complex crochet and knitting patterns that can also be used by us beginner and intermediate knitters with cognitive issues, to provide anchor points. For example, when working a pattern that calls for you to knit a series of rows and then repeat that series, placing a stitch marker (a small safety pin will work just as well) in the final stitch of the final row of that repeat pattern means that if you do forget what row you're working, or if you go wrong and need to unravel your work, you will have a safe point that you can return to, knowing where you are in the pattern. A similar trick that some knitters use in complicated patterns, and that those of us with cognitive impairment or memory issues can take advantage of, is to create a lifeline. This is a piece of thin thread or wool, in a different colour from the yarn you're knitting with, threaded (using a darning needle) through all the stitches on the knitting needle before working that row. Note what row is threaded through and, if all goes hideously wrong, you will have a restore point that you can go back to without being completely lost and having to unravel to the very beginning. Regularly threading a new lifeline reduces the amount of work you risk losing should you get in a muddle.

Crochet tends to grow faster than knitting, using more yarn per stitch, which is worth bearing in mind if you stitch slowly or intermittently. Some consider

Chapter 17

Tunisian crochet, which requires a specific Tunisian crochet hook, to combine the best of both knitting and crochet. Others have found that, despite it producing quicker results, it causes pain that standard crochet doesn't and requires more concentration, so it is clearly a case of finding which works best for you. Tunisian cable hooks hold most of the work for you, so if it's the weight of the work causing pain, this can be a solution.

Another option altogether is nalbinding (or needle binding). This is a Viking technique that predates knitting or crochet and uses a flat needle with an eye large enough to thread chunky yarn through. It is said to be easier on the shoulders, neck and hands and, although stitches take a little longer to work than knitted ones, it tends to grow faster than knitting as each row is about as high as two to three rows of average knitting. Although it is a largely-forgotten craft, books and online instructions for nalbinding are easy to find.

Being able to see the stitches clearly is an issue for any yarn-worker using black or navy yarn, but those of us with chronic illness may have added difficulties, perhaps due to vision issues or light sensitivity affecting how brightly we can tolerate overhead lights. Here, LED light-up crochet hooks and knitting needles come to the rescue. These are particularly useful if you suffer with insomnia and like to crochet at night but share a bed with a partner.

Both knitters and crocheters can benefit from a yarn guide (or yarn splitter if working with different coloured yarns that tangle together). This is worn like a ring at the top of your forefinger, the yarn threaded through to help maintain tension without straining tendons through stretching your finger out. I found a ring amongst my jewellery that conveniently has filigree work I can thread my yarn through for added tension.

Crocheters and knitters with carpal tunnel syndrome, or general aches and soreness in their hands and wrists, often make use of crafters' gloves – compression gloves that aid circulation, reduce swelling and ease discomfort. If repetitive strain is causing painful inflammation, every so often rest your wrist on an ice pack. Remember, too, that you could be unnecessarily adding to the strain by taking the weight of long or heavy projects. When working on these, rest your work on a cushion either on your lap or to the side of you, rather than letting it drag its weight from the needle and thus your wrist.

Knitting machines are an option for those who find the motion of hand knitting or crochet non-negotiable. A circular knitting machine or loom is fairly cheap to buy, and adaptors can be purchased that allow you to power it via an electric screwdriver rather than the standard hand crank. Compatible patterns can be found online as well as tutorials on how to use a circular loom to produce flat pieces of knitting. Rachel is limited in how much hand knitting she can do, due to muscle pain, so she produces the bulk of her jumpers via an electrically powered circular knitting loom. She handcrafts details like the yoke and decorative hem to attach when making the jumper up.

A yarn bowl is a simple tip if you find yourself stuck in bed or on a chair with a runaway ball of wool far from reach on the floor. Any bowl can be used but yarn bowls are designed with a notch or a hole in them for threading the yarn through before beginning work. No matter how much you move around or tug at the yarn, the ball will stay put in the flat-based bowl. Revolving yarn ball holders, that comprise of a flat base with a vertical pole standing on it, to wedge your ball of yarn onto, are another option.

Those of you who like to buy specialist or high-end wool will find that it is sold in hanks or skeins instead of ready-to-use balls or yarn cakes. Using it as it comes isn't an option unless you enjoy regularly untangling a confusion of yarn that resembles the start of a whole new universe. Winding it by hand, slowly and at leisure, can be a satisfyingly meditative act but uses up time and energy that can be saved if you invest in an electric yarn winder or yarn swift.

For those who appreciate the sheep-to-final-product process of spinning one's own yarn, but don't have the physical capability to pedal a traditional spinning wheel, electric spinners are available. They aren't cheap, their cost making them probably only justifiable to the dedicated spinner, unless you purchase one as a group to share, but they certainly take a lot of the effort out of spinning.

And finally, when it comes to blocking knitted or crocheted garments to perfect their shape, knit blockers save some of the time and energy by comprising of up to eight pins, rather than the usual two, in each blocker.

Sewing, beading and felting

A browse of online haberdasheries will reveal a multitude of problem-solving tools. Needle threaders are commonplace in most sewing boxes and especially useful for those affected by tremors. Side-threading needles (sometimes, somewhat more ambitiously, called self-threading needles) are also available. These have a tiny gap at the edge of the eye of the needle so that, by holding the thread with a little tension, you can pull it into the main section of the eye and proceed to sew like normal. Some sewing machines come with an automatic needle threader attachment but, if yours doesn't, a basic needle-threader will serve for the job.

Needle grabbers and pullers are designed to help pull your needle through tough materials like leather or layers of thick upholstery fabric. Those of us with fingers that struggle with gripping needles, or who develop blisters easily, might like to give these a go. The grabbers are a textured pad that you hold between finger and thumb to grasp the needle with, while pullers are little tools that require a pressing action to trigger the device to grasp the needle tightly for you.

Self-threading sewing needles are available.

When it comes to the fiddly action of pinning, easy grip or easy grab pins have larger, shaped heads for ease of use. Meanwhile, sewing clips are an alternative to pins. They look like small bulldog clips and are often used in quilting projects. A magnetic pincushion that you wear around your wrist is a handy accessory and, if you find yourself regularly depositing pins and needles on the floor, a telescopic magnet is a brilliant device for retrieving them without having to bend down.

Cutting fabric, especially if you need many pieces for patchwork or dressmaking, is hard work on the hands and fingers. Even minimal use can leave me with sores, seized joints and general pain. A rotary cutter can bring difficulties of its own, requiring firm pressure to reliably cut through the fabric, but I find that having scissors and my rotary cutter to hand allows me to use whichever is easier in the moment. I sometimes alternate between the two, preventing problems from too much of one kind of movement or friction. When it comes to choosing a rotary cutter, I advise buying a self-locking one that doesn't require you to continuously hold a button down while using it. Pocket rotary cutters are also available for tiny projects or cutting thread. Remember that you will need a cutting board when using one. For the brave and extremely careful amongst you, electric scissors, either battery operated or corded, are available. However, I don't yet know anyone who has trusted themselves with a pair and I like my fingers too much to dare trying them out myself! Electric rotary cutters look marginally less scary…

Quilting gloves are an optional accessory if you want to keep using your faithful old fabric scissors but suffer for doing so. Wearing them reduces friction between the scissors and your fingers as well as any strain on your hands. Rubberised grip dots on the fingertips are also intended to increase control when using pins and threading needles.

While we're talking about cutting fabric, take a lesson from my mistakes and don't be tempted to do this on the floor. A large floor space seems the obvious option when you have vast swathes of fabric to lay out, cut and pin but I advise against it. The extra strain and pain from bending over and stretching will only prevent you from moving on so readily to the next stage of your project. Instead, ensure that you have a surface at the right height for your chair or bedside. A cleared dining table is ideal, especially if it is extendable.

Chapter 17

Even if you usually work in a different room, it's worth the effort of carrying your materials to the dining table to avoid the circulatory and postural abuse inflicted on your body when working on the floor. Even a portable picnic table set up beside the bed, or an ironing board at one of its lowest height settings, can form a temporary work surface at a suitable height. The surface area for you to work on will be acceptable for smaller projects. Draping excess fabric over the back of a chair next to the table will take the weight of the fabric, if you're cutting from large pieces, and prevent it from dragging itself away from you into a heap on the floor.

Sewing machines traditionally operate via a foot pedal but don't worry if you don't have the strength in your legs to operate one, or you need to keep your legs raised. As long as you can sit upright in front of the machine or have an over-bed table that can take the weight of it, you can still use a sewing machine. Just be sure to choose one with the option to sew via a start button that you switch on and off with your finger. You won't need to hold the button while sewing so will still have both hands free for manoeuvring the fabric. In many sewing machines this option is activated when you unplug the foot pedal.

If you are unable to sit upright with your arms held out to work on a table-top sewing machine, a hand-held cordless one could be a solution. It will only sew a basic chain stitch (this looks like regular machine sewing on the top) so fancy stitches are out of the question and, at the end of your row of stitching you must remember to pull your thread through to the back of the fabric, loop it through the final stitch and tie a knot to prevent it unravelling, but as long as you secure it in this way the stitches are strong and reliable. Don't be tempted by the very cheap mini handheld sewing machines that work not via batteries but by the manual action of pressing it down like a staple gun. These rarely work reliably, leading to inevitable disappointment.

Appliqué and small pieces of crazy patchwork can be achieved using a fabric glue stick. Using glue instead of pinning or tacking and meticulously sewing reserves your capabilities for the more fun, decorative stitches. Iron-on double-sided adhesive fabric, such as Bondaweb, is also useful. If you are unable to lift the weight of an iron, mini irons are available specifically for crafting, or a travel iron may be manageable. An alternative to an iron, for small areas or seams, is a set of hair straighteners, although bear in mind that the temperature is not adjustable so unsuitable for particularly heat-sensitive fabric.

Hand embroidery, cross-stitch and tapestry would seem to be such gentle pastimes and yet my body manages to struggle even with something so sedate. It turns out my left arm particularly objects to the position I ask it to maintain (inner forearm facing sideways rather downwards) when holding my work. I was thrilled when I learned about embroidery stands that hold, via a clamp, your embroidery hoop for you. Mine is attached to a flat stand that I sit on, enabling me to angle the arm of the stand to hold my work at a comfortable height above my lap. Floor-standing embroidery stands and cross-stitch frames are also available.

In conjunction with my embroidery stand, I use a magnifying glass with an inbuilt LED light. Again, this is on an angle-poise stand and, by having it positioned between my work and my eyes I can sew tiny stitches without either bending my neck or having to lift my hands up closer to my face. This way I may look like I am using enough equipment to perform minor surgery but at least I can keep my arms and head resting against cushions as I sew. Floor-standing illuminated magnifying glasses are available, as are the less cumbersome type that go around your neck, like a giant necklace, with a ledge to prop it at an angle against your chest as you work.

The more artistic among you probably enjoy designing your own projects and may not have considered buying mass-produced kits. However, with the materials pre-measured and supplied with specific instructions, the energy you would have spent on researching and prepping is provided by someone else, leaving you free to sew. 'But,' I hear some of you cry, 'I enjoy making original pieces and playing with my own ideas'. I know. I also know that there is a time and place for incorporating other people's offerings into our creativity and that, when not well enough to contemplate a whole project from scratch, a pre-prepared kit can enable us to make something rather than nothing. The rest of you are probably shaking your heads in bewilderment at why we wouldn't avail ourselves of the beautiful kits out there. Downloadable embroidery and cross-stitch patterns are also available if you have the threads and fabric but not the capability (or inclination) to draw your own designs.

Adding **beads** to your sewing, or working on a purely beaded piece, is fiddly work not helped by poor hand-eye coordination, shakes, tremors or the uneven surface of a bed or lap. My invaluable assistant here is my beading mat. Very cheap and made from microfibre, its texture stops dropped beads, or those spread out to sift through, from rolling away. As for the teeny-tiny eyes on beading needles – if you don't require a sharp point for penetrating fabric, perhaps threading beads together for jewellery making – wire beading needles have a flexible eye that can be opened wide to insert the thread and squeezed shut to pass through the tiniest of beads.

Another textile craft I've embarked on, only to find that my muscles weren't as enthusiastic as my mind, is **wet-felting**. The general advice is to either put your wool rovings on a sushi rolling mat or sandwich it between layers of bubble wrap or netting to aid friction, but much repetitive rubbing is still required to successfully felt the wool. You don't need great dexterity but some stamina is necessary. Felt-rolling machines can be purchased but you probably won't want to spend in excess of a thousand pounds. Instead, when wet-felting small pieces such as brooches or flowers, an electric toothbrush will impart the motion for you as you glide it over the surface of your work. I still found this took too long for me and required more energy than I could provide, so I invited an orbital sander (sans sandpaper) to the table. I could only use it for a short time due to both its weight and the vibrations, but it did enable me to have a go at wet-felting. Now, obviously, you and I both know that nobody who values their life would ever mix electricity and water so, for this reason, ONLY use a wireless sander and place it inside a couple of securely sealed carrier bags before use to prevent any soapy splashes causing problems.

Another form of felting that requires repetitive movement is **needle-felting**. No water is involved in this process – just wool rovings and a barbed felting needle that you repeatedly punch in and out and in and out to felt the wool together. A felting tool (also called a handle or holder) that several felting needles can be slotted into at once will speed up your work and, being fatter than the handle on a single needle, may be easier to hold. The ones that hold seven needles won't provide the accuracy you may desire to create intricate designs but they are handy for larger, less precise areas. Some felting tools allow you to choose whether to insert one, two or three needles at any time. The ultimate energy saving tool for this craft, however, is a handheld electric dry felting machine.

Drawing and painting

Wide-bodied and ergonomic pens and paint brushes can be bought if you have difficulty gripping standard-sized ones. Alternatively, a search on the internet will offer up various pen and pencil grippers that can be taken on and off your existing drawing and painting tools, and searching for arthritis aids will bring up many suggestions.

There are also several DIY solutions. Some people suggest holding the paint brush or pencil with putty in your hand. The putty will mould to the shape of your hand and assist your grip. For a more permanent solution on a particular tool, Sugru (an air-hardening adhesive silicone rubber that comes in small sachets) can be moulded in a comfortable shape around the handle, or you could do what has temporarily worked for me in the past and use Blu-tac. Another option, this time for a chunkier aid, is to make a hole through a tennis ball, squishy stress ball or egg-shaped makeup sponge, large enough to insert your paintbrush handle but small enough to firmly grip it for you.

Chapter 17

The ball can then be held in the palm of your hand, allowing your fingers to take it easy.

Creativity is a great problem solver so think laterally and you may come up with your own device for holding your tools with greater ease. I have seen a macramé sleeve for paint brush handles that one woman made out of an old phone charger cable. She glued the ends down to secure them in place and then slipped the sleeve onto the paintbrush.

When confined to bed or the sofa, painting becomes a trickier activity. Lap easels are an option but remember that holding arms above the height of the heart exerts extra stress on the cardiovascular system. Where possible, rest your arms on pillows. And then there's all that colourful liquid combined with bumpy cushions, uneven surfaces and your favourite soft furnishings: a recipe for mess if I were involved. Non-spill paint pots may enable less perilous painting in these circumstances. Another solution is a set of aqua or refillable watercolour brushes. These are paint brushes that incorporate a water reservoir in the handle of the brush itself.

To create a painted effect without having to purchase or mix up and clean away paints, Sharon says, 'Something I love doing in bed is using water-based felt pens/marker pens. Use a small brush and a little water over it and it blends. I sometimes use colour pencil on them when they're dry.' Watercolour pencils (that can be used as normal colouring pencils or combined with water to create a watercolour effect), blend-able watercolour brush pens and acrylic paint pens are all less messy, easier to handle and quicker to tidy away alternatives that may satisfy your urge when unable to use traditional paints. A bonus of acrylic and other water-based pens is that they don't give off the fumes that some people react to when using pens containing alcohol.

Many chronically ill and disabled artists are availing themselves of what technology can offer, finding digital art welcomes them back into a world of creativity. From free collaging apps (Dada is fun and easy to navigate) to digital painting, there are ways to explore visual arts without all the usual paraphernalia.

'I fell in love with what I was seeing achieved in Procreate by other artists,' says Rachel F. 'I'm so excited to learn more and create more, especially when too tired and mal-coordinated to dare using real watercolours in bed!' While using Procreate on an iPad does seem to be the most widely appreciated of the digital art apps, there is much enthusiasm for some of the many free drawing apps on both Apple and Android touch-screen devices (Fresco, HiPaint, Illustrator, Infinite Painter, Krita, Paper and Sketchbook being some of the most recommended, at the time of writing). These can all be used with your finger, choosing from a multitude of virtual brushes, pens and pencils to alter the effect, but some find a stylus or Apple pencil improves their results. Online tutorials abound to acclimatise you to digital art and guide you through the process. If you're not sure how the difference in feel between a screen and the paper that you're more familiar with will affect your art, paper-feel screen protectors are available. These give the sensation of drawing on a more traditional surface and provide greater control over the marks made.

Whatever medium you choose, it's all too easy to feel frustrated when weak or shaking hands prevent you from creating what you envisaged. Perhaps, instead of feeling dejected, you might explore the patterns, marks and images you can create when you welcome the shakes and wobbles instead of attempting to curb them. The result might look naïve to you while still being a valid creative outlet. You may even decide you prefer the freer, more relaxed appearance of what emerges. Paula Knight was a professional illustrator for 15 years. She now requires full-time care but has found ways to integrate art into her severely confined life, one of which adapts Paul Klee's method of 'taking a line for a walk'. 'I've taken a few lines for a lie down while bedridden,' she says. 'Pencil drawings were made by resting a sketchpad on my diaphragm and trying not to lose my

Explore the patterns, marks and images you create when you welcome the shakes and wobbles instead of attempting to curb them.

grip on the pencil. The drawings could be considered kinaesthetic – they are traces of body and breath – evidence of life.'

The written word

As with painting, refillable aqua pens can be a way to avoid messy spillages when practising brush calligraphy. Fill one with ink and you needn't have an open ink pot just waiting to be knocked over. And just as with drawing, writing can be eased with an ergonomic pen, Arthwriter hand aid or one of the many styles of pen/pencil grips.

Tremors that make your writing illegible can be compensated for with a weighted pen or a weighted grip aid. You can create your own weighted pencil by pilfering some hex nuts from a toolbox and sliding these onto your pencil with an elastic band at each end to prevent them from slipping off.

If you write lying down with a tilted surface above you but find pen ink drains away from the nib, zero-gravity space pens that work at any angle are an option. Meanwhile, wireless keyboards will allow the prone writer to have their screen and keyboard in different places so they can see what they're typing while keeping their arms supported lower down. Ergonomic keyboards or wrist rests may reduce hand and wrist pain when typing.

Speech to text software is great for getting basic ideas and sentences down, even if you aren't comfortable finely honing your writing through speech alone. I alternate handwriting, dictation, using a Swype keyboard on my phone screen (this uses far less energy than tapping out individual letters) and typing on my laptop as my body allows.

Zero-gravity space pens work at any angle, even lying down with a tilted surface above you.

Smartphones, tablets and Word documents come with an inbuilt dictation option that allows you to easily move between speech and typing. Dictation software, apps and websites offering free-speech/

voice-to-text functions are also worth investigating to see which you get along with best. Google Docs can be used on any device, allowing you to pick up where you left off when moving between your phone and a laptop. Otter is a well-rated app particularly worth a mention here. As well as being an easy-to-use and accurate dictation device, it can transcribe (in real time) online meetings, interviews, talks and podcasts, making note-taking a far less energy-consuming task.

Even when speaking to your device, reading back the text on the screen for editing purposes can be a problem for those with light sensitivity or who suffer from eye strain. Give your eyes a break as often as possible by closing them or looking away into the distance when dictating. Reserve limited screen time for when you need to read what you've written and observe whether some screens are easier on your eyes than others. Despite a phone screen being smaller, I suffer fewer symptoms from viewing text on a mobile phone than on a laptop.

Whatever device you use, do remember to turn the screen brightness down to the level that is most comfortable for you and, if a more yellow tint (instead of the blue-infused light that glares from screens) is more tolerable, activate the night-shift or night-light mode. Night mode can be set on laptops, tablets and smart phones for whatever hours of the day you choose so don't be fooled by its name into thinking it's only a perk for night writers and bedtime researchers.

Aside from the mechanics of how we get the words down, a writer's primary material is the words themselves. When brain fog, fatigue or pain are clouding thoughts and concealing even the most basic nouns and adjectives, we are left wondering how we'll ever produce anything worth reading or listening to. Rather than railing against this difficulty, can the brain fog sometimes serve you? Mixed up words, spoonerisms and confused phrases can be harnessed as humorous, poignant and unique descriptions. Avoiding clichés and breaking away from the obvious are something writers so often struggle with and yet here is your brain accidentally nudging you in an original direction. Just writing these linguistic tangles down as a (perhaps illustrated) foggy dictionary is one way of utilising them. 'Glass curtain' (window), 'bird leaves' (feathers) and 'plug yourself in' (put on your seat belt) are all ways my weary brain has attempted to liven up the English language. Perhaps, at times, this symptom can be used as an aid in itself.

A handy piece of kit is a fridge poetry set. These sets comprise of hundreds of magnetised words that are great to play with when ideas are eluding you. They encourage unusual linguistic connections, based on the random words in front of you, instigating lines of poetry or story titles that wouldn't otherwise have occurred to your beleaguered brain. Used on a magnetic board instead of a fridge, this creativity assistant can accompany you wherever you have to park your body. Extra words can be included by sticking paper to self-adhesive magnetic tape, writing your chosen words on the paper, and then cutting the magnetic tape to size. Cut-out poetry, where you snip words and short phrases from magazine and newspaper articles or old books that nobody minds you destroying, and jiggling them around on a tray, achieves the same purpose.

Another way to be creative with the written word without having to think up whole sentences from scratch is blackout poetry. Typically, you'd pick a newspaper or magazine page and use a marker pen to black out all the words apart from the ones you want to remain visible to be read as a poem. This technique can be updated by screenshotting online text and using the mark-up function in a photo-editing app to block out unwanted words. And, of course, this technique needn't just be for creating poetry. Flash fiction, micro-fiction, opening paragraphs, titles, thought provocations and exuberant nonsense can all be generated via this method. By offering your mind a loose path to follow, the pressure to pluck sentences from the depths of thick fog is diminished, leaving you freer to discover what's already right there with you.

Pottery and sculpting

Unless there are local classes that you're well enough to attend, or you are lucky enough to have access to a kiln, pottery may have felt out of your creative range but there are options.

Air-drying clay is relatively cheap and comes in white, natural clay and terracotta colours. It doesn't require water or slip and, once hardened at room temperature, is ready for painting. It can even be used on a potter's wheel and, before you ask me where you're supposed to find a potter's wheel around your home, let me tell you that mini electric pottery wheels are available at not too great a cost online. Yes, this information excited me, too!

Another alternative to traditional clay is polymer clay. This requires baking in a standard kitchen oven to harden. You can choose either plain white and decorate it yourself (acrylic paints can be applied either before or after baking) or purchase individual pre-coloured blocks that you combine (marbling them together is effective). Liquid polymer mixed with powdered pigment (strongly pigmented powder eyeshadow can also be used) and applied to plain white unbaked polymer clay will stick to the unhardened clay, emerging from the oven with a glazed ceramic effect. Substitute powdered pigment with oven-safe metallic pigment powder and your piece will resemble metal. Meanwhile, liquid polymer can be poured into oven-proof silicone moulds to create intricately shaped pieces for you to paint.

Photography

Staying for a moment with visual arts, photography is accessible to many of us now that camera phones have become so advanced, but the dedicated photographers among you will probably yearn for more professional equipment that is still light enough to hold with relative ease. The lesser weight of a mirrorless camera, as opposed to the popular and cheaper DSLR cameras, may make this worth the extra cost for you.

As well as weight, a primary factor for me when choosing a camera is that it has a stabilisation feature to offset the wobble in my hands. Image/lens/optical stabilisation are all different names for the same thing whereas sensor stabilisation functions differently. Very simply summarised for our purposes here, the latter results in a lighter camera whereas the former is better for long telephoto images.

Not having to hold arms aloft and steady while waiting for the perfect shot opens more photographic opportunities for the chronically ill photographer. To this end, a mini tripod with legs that swivel and bend to attach to branches, poles and bars, or balance on surfaces as uneven as rocks, a lap or your bed is a useful accessory. These can be used with cameras or smartphones, adaptors being available for different equipment. There are a few lightweight flexible tripod stands on the market, GorillaPod and Octopus being ones that I've seen recommended.

Music

Guitars, mandolins and ukuleles all lend themselves to being played sat down, which is a distinct advantage for chronically ill musicians. Small Celtic or lyre harps are also perfect for playing sat on a chair or bed as their size is designed for placing on your lap. If brain fog makes learning to play these too taxing, a zither (also known as a lap harp) is a lovely option. The strings are on a small board that you lay horizontally on your lap, meaning you can keep your arms lowered while playing it. Music can be made via improvisation or by learning the notes of the strings. Some lap harps come with song sheets of familiar tunes that you slide between the base board and the strings to see which strings to pluck in which order.

For the piano lovers amongst you, an electric keyboard can be set up at your bedside or even played over your lap if you're happy with a reduced octave range. You may find that the keys are easier to press than traditional piano keys. Even smaller scale is a thumb piano or kalimba – a westernised version of the traditional Zimbabwean instrument, the mbira. It is a small, light piano-style percussion instrument that you can hold in your lap.

Wind instruments can be heavy or awkward to hold as well as requiring precise embouchure that can be very tiring on facial muscles, but there are some easier options. Many of us associate recorders with screechy primary school practice but they can sound beautiful when played well. Treble (also known as alto) recorders have a deeper more mellow sound than descant recorders so may be easier on the ear for those with sensitivity to higher sounds. A traditional wooden Native American-style flute has a lovely sound and is played more like a recorder than the western flute. Similarly, it requires less rigid embouchure and arms can be held less aloft than when using a side-played flute. Other wind or mouth-played instruments that are light to hold are the harmonica (mouth organ) and jaw harp. The latter is a very rudimentary instrument but fun to play.

If drumming is your thing, small djembe drums or a Celtic bodhran can both be played in your usual seat or even from bed.

Musicians who struggle with sound sensitivity may find that Ear Loops enable them to enjoy their instrument, even playing along with others, without being overwhelmed by the volume. These are a type of ear plug that reduce background and peripheral noise while still allowing you to clearly hear the instrument you're playing or the person you're conversing with. By reducing extraneous sound, the brain has less to filter and hyperacuity can become less of a problem.

Singing is a joyful solo experience but even more powerful when voices work together. Those of you who are lifted by the magic that results from group singing might like to consider online choirs. There are many to be found via an internet search and location is no object when everyone attending is online. As well as events attended at a synchronised time, there is the option of collaborating with others at your own convenience, with all contributions being digitally combined to create a harmonious performance. Game Choir is one such initiative that simultaneously raises money for Special Effect, a charity that helps provide specialist gaming equipment for young people with physical disabilities.

Staying with digital musicianship, the Clarion is a recently developed instrument to look out for that is designed to be accessible to disabled musicians. It is played via digital software using any part of the body, including the eyes.

Gardening

For all you creative gardeners with reduced movement or limited access to beds of the herbaceous kind, all is not lost. Tending to plants without stretching or bending is made more possible with telescopic-handled trowels, forks, rakes and weeders, long-handled secateurs and reaching/grabber tools. Conversely, tools that normally have long handles, such as hoes, can be bought as hand hoes, or forked hand hoes, to suit seated gardening.

Ergonomic, rotating anvil secateurs are designed to be lighter, easier and more comfortable to use than standard secateurs. Easi-grip garden tools take the strain off your wrist (a compatible arm cuff to attach them to is also available), while upright handled tools may be more comfortable to hold if you have limited movement in your wrists. Thumb cutters, meanwhile, are a little blade on a silicone thimble worn on your thumb for deadheading flowers without the need for secateurs. They come with a safety sleeve for your forefinger to prevent cutting yourself when applying pressure.

Those of you with a larger garden than you have stamina to walk around or stand in for any length of time might find relief in the form of a gardening seat on wheels, or a wheeled tool cart with a seat on top. A garden kneeler is designed to be used either as a stool to sit on or turned upside down to kneel on the ground on the underside of the seat while using the upturned legs as supports to lift yourself up from the ground.

Raised beds in a garden will bring gardening to a seat-friendly height and save you from bending down or getting stuck on the ground. Alternatively, wheelchair-accessible wooden planters and collections of pots on tables, stands and in window boxes are much easier to manage than a sprawling garden, especially if you either leave adequate space for a wheelchair or have outdoor seats to sit on while watering and tending.

If you are unable to regularly give your plants the attention they need, automatic watering systems and self-watering systems can be bought (or simple DIY ones made from old water bottles) to save them from dehydrating.

Terrariums, bonsai collections, indoor plants and flower displays are all ways to interact creatively with nature while restricted to indoor living.

But what about a gardener without access to outside space? Consider yourself a gardener of the indoor variety. Terrariums, bonsai collections, creative arrangements of indoor plants and flower displays are all ways to satisfy the desire to interact creatively with the colours and shapes of nature while restricted to indoor living. Air plants only need watering during spring and summer and, even then, only once a week, making them one of the easier plants for the ill to care for. They can be displayed in all manner of unusual ways: suspended from hooks, placed inside glass jars, even glued to pieces of driftwood!

 Suggested creative exercise
Tools of the trade

Take stock of the equipment your chosen craft requires and be realistic about physical issues you may have with it. Evaluate how you can better get along with it and any adaptations you could make. Investigate alternative tools. Research aids for the disabled and the elderly. Find what is available for fulltime and professional artists and crafters. While you may not fall into these categories, your needs could benefit from more comfortable or time-saving devices.

Create-ability at a glance

- Online tutorials are the next best thing to attending an in-person class.
- Use rhymes and other memory aids to remember complicated sequences when learning a new skill.
- Make use of any disability aids that could help, preferably before they become vital.
- Aids designed for the elderly can provide assistance and comfort.
- Investigate professional craft tools and equipment that could make engagement in your hobby easier for you.
- Research around your craft to see what similar alternatives may be more accessible to you.
- Use technology to assist you so that you can put more energy into the creative side of your craft.

Chapter 18
Fallow times and beyond

Just as each day requires a night off before the next dawn, so we have our rhythms, whether we like them or nor. What we call fallow times might be exactly what our creativity needs – a period of refreshing not just our body but our inspiration as well. In fact, 'Resting is essential for creativity to flow,' observes Jabeen, a painter with chronic illness. It's helpful to hold onto this knowledge when our body insists on us taking time out. Perhaps a bonus of our daily existence quietening so much is that we can hear what our muse has been whispering all along.

Long periods of inactivity and enforced rest become all too familiar to the chronically ill, revisiting us periodically, if not grindingly regularly. While frustrating and often boring, these times can still be used to creative advantage. When the body is constantly busy, the brain is having to process all that is going on. Too often we let the world around us glide off our retinas or become a hum in the background. Our times of rest and stillness, of what feel like removal from the world, can be embraced as periods of attentive awareness to the moment. With senses on high alert and movements slowed down we can respond with curiosity to our immediate experience, pondering what it is about sounds, objects, textures, and sensations that appeals to or jars with us.

Being creative doesn't require continuously constructing tangible output. Inspirationally and physically, there is a fine line between healthy endeavour and unhealthy struggle. When frustrated by creative inactivity, remain open to the ever-present sources of possibility without pushing or pulling for ideas or motivation that aren't forthcoming. In the same vein, striving for activity that isn't advisable is more likely to set your health back and bring further disappointment than if you accept the reality of this moment. Trust in the forward motion of baby steps or even the battery-charging power of total inertia.

Resist forcing yourself to create what isn't ready to be brought into being. By craning your neck to foretell the end of a project you've had to put on hold, or a loose idea that you don't seem able to develop, perhaps you are looking in an unhelpful direction. The path to the horizon often dips and deviates from expectation, even curving out of view. Allow your creativity to follow the same natural flow, and focus for now on what is within reach. How can you work creatively with that?

Expanding our definition of creativity

When our bodies prevent us from engaging with the kind of activities we aim for, it is an opportunity to be more generous about how we define our creativity. Doodling freely, choosing hues for colouring in, journaling, freestyling random word associations; the décor we surround ourselves with, the language we use in our heads, the awareness with which we experience our senses... We can support our creative selves without being explicitly productive.

Be generous about how you define creativity.

Anna B writes fiction when her chronic illness allows. At other times she does whatever her body can manage to express her creativity. 'Scribbling and doodling stuff I'll just stick in the bin afterwards can be good. I quite like having a file of collage stuff just to randomly stick together – not to show anyone! I still have a bunch of paper horses I made years ago with moveable legs and tails. I was just playing around, each one weirdly decorated however I felt and totally unrealistic, but it felt satisfying having a growing herd.'

When sketching partial images, contemplating a collection of colours with nowhere substantial to land, or turning stranded words over in my mind, either without the health or the inspiration to take them further, it is all too

Chapter 18

easy to feel unworthy of being considered creative. The fear is that if we don't imminently incorporate our thoughts into a fully formed idea we have failed, but this is an illusion based on the expectation of quantifiable results. Don't shut down recognition of yourself as creative just because it's not coming together in the instant. We are still creative beings, but we are in receptive and digestive mode. We are biding our time, gathering and absorbing by osmosis.

Be observant in your stillness. Allow your senses to recognise and interpret creativity wherever they settle, be that the design of a mundane object, print on a bedspread, textures of a cushion cover, bare branches outside a window, rain on a pane of glass, steam rising from a hot drink, dust motes in a shaft of sunlight. Our brain is learning to exist as creatively as our collaboration with the moment can encourage.

It may even be that your lack of ideas, or energy to bring them into being, forms a creative response in itself. The following is one tangible result of my own frustration:

> Soap bubble ideas
>   pop
>   pop
> pop
> Die in my wiped-out mind.

Become a curator of creativity. Gaze on art cards and pictures from magazines, drape textural scarves where you can touch them, eat from a beautiful plate or bowl, treat yourself to items handmade by others. Collect art and craft and photography books, simply enjoying their spines lined up on a bookshelf, knowing the covers are safekeeping the contents for when you can dive in. Dip in and out of literature (whether spoken or on the page) just to enjoy the rhythms of sentences, with no pressure to concentrate on large tracts of text. Let your surroundings remind you, even in your dormant times, of your deepest self and your wildest pleasures.

My piano may not feel herself played for many months (sometimes years) at a time but she's always there, faithfully reminding me that she's ready for my return. I change the sheet music on the stand when it suits me, even if I'm not up to playing it. Just knowing it's there, in the open, is of comfort. I am a music maker, no matter how long since I last pressed the keys.

A musician who makes no sound, an illustrator who draws only in their mind's eye, a bedbound dancer, a garden designer with no outside space… We are still our creative selves. Immerse yourself, however you can, in influences and aesthetic expression that remind you of this.

Creativity's silent partner

The author Anthony Horowitz considers his readers (or audiobook devourers) to be co-creators of the novels he writes, using their own imagination to create worlds out of his words. The poet Naomi Shihab Nye agrees when she reminds us that listening to the spoken word is not a passive act but a participatory one. After all, art thrives on an audience to respond to it. Involve yourself by absorbing rather than doing. Allow yourself to be a silent partner with creativity. If you're able to take this act one step further by learning lines of poetry off by heart to recite to yourself, then you will have them with you even when unable to read or listen to the words.

When I shared a mixed media collage online that highlighted the gap between my abilities and my desires, Marion, a chronically ill friend responded, 'Love that you used mascara. Made me think of a tear-stained face with black streaks running down cheeks. For all that we mourn.' I had simply used mascara because it was accessible to me, and I liked the marks that a mascara wand could make. Marion's interpretation hadn't occurred to me, but it added another layer to what I had been trying to convey. I thanked her for her contribution to the piece.

Your response to another's creativity unites you with the original artist in a co-creation that spans space and time. This is valuable, whether you voice it or not. Monica Michelle is an illustrator, novelist and podcaster with Ehlers-Danlos syndrome. She advises her listeners to be an audience to all that they can be, especially when anything else is beyond their means. Creative offerings gather more life when they have an audience and, sometimes, creativity by proxy is the best answer to the question 'what can I do?' John, mostly housebound with chronic illness, does exactly this with film scores and classical music. When held indoors, away from the country views he so loves, he closes his eyes and listens to pastoral suites by Vaughan-Williams, collaborating with the music to disappear off into bucolic pictures in his mind.

We know from results in places of care and the workplace, as well as clinical studies, that music, artwork and scenic views can bestow beneficial effects and activate reward circuitry in the brain. For creative people incapacitated by illness, the need for aesthetic comforts is even greater. When the painter Turner was nearing the end of his life, and illness prevented him from producing much artwork, he returned to his cottage with the views of the Thames and the wide skies that he adored. He wasn't painting but he was allowing his mind to absorb and process the scenery, in memory of the scenes he once reproduced on canvas. For him, this must surely have been a diluted, yes, but passively creative act.

As your body gains nourishment from times of rest, so too can your inner artist.

As your body gains nourishment from times of rest so too can your inner artist. For now, just for now, taking time to enjoy the colour palette of the sky outside, of vegetables on a plate, a stash of yarn, a paintbox, or someone else's artistic output can be enough. Engage and enjoy whichever senses and offerings are comfortably available to you.

Cultivating imagination

Simply imagining is one of the most creative things we can do, and not just as the precursor for physical projects. 'I went to America today, on the wide wings of imagination, to a place in the mountains,' Sarah-Louise Jordan declares from her bed. Some days her symptoms are so severe that even imaginative travel is beyond her but when she returns from the darkest places, it is her inner world that keeps her going: 'It's been a while since my daydreams have been a clear, deep lagoon that I can swim in. Things are dastardly right now and it is all very painful, but it's lovely to be able to leap off the rocks in my imagination. I'm grateful to be able to frolic in a place where the light dances on the surface of the water and the ripples that spread out from each thought can lead me into every kind of adventure.'

When my mind is strong enough to be searching out interesting ways to occupy itself but not able to stay with extended thoughts, I sometimes exercise my creativity by simulating an exercise taught to art students. They are given a large piece of paper, told to choose an object and then draw it in as many different guises or scenarios as they can come up with. I have seen one student choose an electricity pylon as their subject, depicting it, amongst other things, skipping, decorated like a festive tree with fairy lights, and holding up a washing line with another pylon. Another chose a carrot, one of the pictures being a visual pun on the gardening concept of a vegetable bed. I forego the drawing part of this process and test my creative thinking by seeing how many images I can summon in my mind's eye. Drifting in and out of concentration, you might surprise yourself with the creative ideas you conjure.

Even within times of being too unwell to make art, we can usually still gaze on things, however momentarily, with the observation of an active artist. Let your eyes rest on the petals of cut flowers, a bowl of fruit, the folds and creases of a blanket, and imagine how you could represent them in different media. Examine the shades of colour and lines of shadow as if you were embarking on an artistic interpretation. The art here is in the use of your mind, no matter how fleetingly. It is not an exercise in talent but a creative way to pass ill time and honour your intrinsic creativity.

Listening to snippets of world music or foreign languages is another way to cultivate inner creativity. Explore how the rhythms and cadences affect you. Close your eyes and investigate the patterns that form and mutate in your mind, as well as the way your body physically responds.

For years Whitney didn't have the luxury of enjoying his senses. Due to the severity of his ME he had to lie in the dark with as little stimulation as possible, but his creative nature would not be thwarted. Indeed, it was interludes of following his imagination that kept him going. Able now to write about this time he says, 'I let my mind wander. I usually thought about making things … I also thought about art projects in depth, of course. I lived for that time of daydreaming … and somehow made a sort of life out of it.' When your existence is monopolised by surviving the basics of living, that is all that matters. Outward expression of creativity is for another time. But know, just like Whitney, that it still resides within you underneath the harshness of the long moment.

And when those long moments are clogged with thoughts, fears or frustrations that are taking up more of your brain power than you'd like, exacerbated by having to refrain from physical or sensory stimulation, a craft-related mental game can help you to settle on something more relaxing. Visualising yourself slowly raking the sand of a Zen garden into pleasing patterns can be an especially soothing way to occupy yourself with the activity of soothing your mind into a state of abstract order. Or how about repeatedly filling the easel of your mind with a hand-lettered mantra or affirmation in varying colours and designs? Similar imagery can be employed with the medium of your choice: sorting, smoothing, erasing, weeding or unpicking; moulding, pruning, arranging and painting a calmer mental state.

Patient preparations

I crave physical movement when having to rest for endless hours. Even tiny physical actions related to crafting can fulfil that need for motion and involvement in hobbies and so, lying flat in bed, I like to pretend I'm playing the piano. Scales, arpeggios and finger exercises, hearing music in my head, or listening to recordings of music that I can play in better times, I imagine I'm playing along. Sometimes I can move my fingers as if I were at the piano, other times I just visualise the actions, feeling each finger twitch slightly when their turn comes. I also satisfy this urge by improvising sentences or reciting verse in my mind that I imagine typing out on a keyboard. Visualising physical movement activates the same neural pathways as when you perform the actual motion. While this means that you may need to limit how vividly and regularly you perform such activities in your mind, it is a great transition exercise so that when you return to whatever task you're imagining you will feel familiar with the movements.

Anna M recognises her body's need to shut down at times. She has learnt the simplicity, if not the ease, of the situation, knowing that there is no point in berating her body for not being able to do what she'd like. Instead, she recognises that she can use this inactive time to allow her well of inspiration to refill, so that she's ready to get started when her body catches up with her urges. 'When I can't create, I don't. I am just surviving and waiting it out. I look at other people's work, look for inspiration and make things in my head for when the crash is over and I can start bringing them to life.'

It's perfectly okay to do nothing, absorb nothing new and think no coherent thoughts when resting. There is no obligation to have your creativity button always switched on, no pressure for output or improvement. But when the particularly difficult days drag on, and your mind is more eager than your body, times of imposed stillness lend themselves to theoretically learning new methods and techniques.

Anna B has her own tried and tested ways of getting through the harder days. 'In bad patches,' she recalls, 'I can't do crafty stuff at all. Sometimes I watch tutorials and people making online.' Anna's viewing choice isn't uncommon in the ill community. Many find it soothing to watch artists at work and crafters talking us through techniques and projects. YouTube and other viewing platforms abound with people sharing the processes and development of their work. This form of slow TV tends to be less taxing than television dramas or films and can be watched repeatedly, both for the pure pleasure of vicarious creativity and for the information to gradually lodge in even a severely fatigued brain.

Your body may not want to practise today, but you can prepare the way for when you do feel well enough. You might even save yourself wasted energy or expense by learning that what you thought you were missing out on isn't for you after all. Watching crafts that you don't have the inclination to take part in can also impart tips and ideas to cross-reference to your own areas of interest. During these fallow times, when accomplished projects are beyond you, build up banks of ideas to draw upon and pitfalls to avoid.

Lay down further groundwork by recording whatever ideas stumble into your periphery. File away feelings, phrases, snapshots and vignettes that can be retrieved when another flash of inspiration or stronger health facilitates their use. Take the tiniest seeds of ideas and, rather than dismissively blowing them aside or promising yourself you will remember them later (hear your muse laugh as she carries them elsewhere at such a suggestion!), plant them immediately in an ever-present notebook, a treasure box, your phone's photo reel, or a voice note.

Gather and grow a fertile library for the future you to access and build upon. And let it be. You can revisit this resource later, whenever you feel inclined, and see what you come up with hours, days, weeks or even years from now. Your current task is simply to let life, as quickly or slowly as it desires, fill your internal cabinet of curiosities.

> *Take the tiniest seeds of ideas and plant them immediately in an ever-present notebook, a treasure box, your phone's photo reel, or a voice note.*

It doesn't matter how occasional or spare these deposits in your creativity bank are – an isolated image, interesting word, colour cut from a glossy magazine, or new technique without a project to attach it to. Even if they seem insignificant on their own, something you come up with or encounter in years to come may combine perfectly with one of them. In the meantime, this collection becomes a reminder of your appreciations and intentions: your creative spirit.

Recently, when too unwell to engage in crafting, an idea came to me of miniature hand-sewn archetype dolls. This concept has lain inside me for a little while now. I feel an urge to manifest these mythic companion characters but am still not up to embarking on the process. Perhaps paper doll versions will be a way of developing the concept as I wait for greater strength. Perhaps this will be enough. Will they ever be stitched into being? I don't know, but for the moment I'm enjoying lining them up on a little wooden shelf on the edge of my mind, taking them down periodically to design more imaginary details before setting them back for safe keeping. Whether it is their safe keeping or mine I'm not entirely sure. We are in half-lit worlds, guarding and dreaming each other's existence. I wonder what they are visualising for me.

Engaging playfully with creative activities

As you begin to recover from a prolonged period of stasis you may not feel ready to leap into a full-blown project. It takes time to acclimatise to a shifted circumstance, both mentally and physically. At this tender stage of re-building a functional level of health we must be extra careful. And so, as with my idea of paper precursor dolls, we ponder what won't set our body back into a relapse as well as how to guide our mind back into creative confidence.

In that liminal space between devilishly heavy symptoms and a more dynamic existence, be especially relaxed with yourself about what you can achieve. You might have a workbook that you try out ideas in or scraps of fabric to play with stitches on. Ease yourself in without any intent to take the work further, gently exercising your creativity while your physical muscles remember how it feels to handle the tools.

Chapter 18

When I'm only up to a small activity that requires little concentration or commitment, I like to re-organise my craft equipment. I tidy a lone drawer that has become jumbled, sort through a pencil case to rekindle my connection with its contents, or wind ribbons and lace trims that have snuck across to converse with each other while I had my eyes shut. I usually have hand-me-down tangles of yarn or skeins of wool stored away for future use and find it soothing to prop myself up and slowly, very slowly, untangle and wind yarn. The softer the yarn and more appealing the colour, the more therapeutic the action. The knots don't stress me as I have no aim to sort them out quickly. It's just something to do with my hands while my head and arms rest on pillows. I can pick it up for a few minutes at a time, leaving it again for as long as necessary, and know that I'm contributing to a distant creation.

This may seem like procrastination but it feeds the creative habit. It touches that part of me that needs to interact with colour and possibility. Creating order in this way can be comforting amidst the unpredictability of chronic illness and will often result in playing with what I find or remembering something I acquired some time ago but never got around to using. If I'm lucky I will discover things side by side that I wouldn't have deliberately combined and my mind, having been distanced from creative assuredness by incapacity, switches back into experimental mode, toying with directions I can explore.

To re-ignite faded motivation or to fill the gap between *I'm just focusing on being able to turn over in bed right now* and *Look! I made a thing!* allow yourself this freedom of play. Instead of reminding yourself of all the reasons why you can't engage with your craft as fully as you'd like, do what you can, however seemingly insignificant. The author Susanna Clarke recognises that her method for writing the novel *Piranesi* while chronically ill didn't conform to any traditional advice that authors are guided to follow. She advises others struggling with energy-limiting illness to only write as they are able, without pressure to be doing what they think they should. The same goes for anything you feel inclined to try. Simply do what you can to have fun.

If you don't have the energy to work with oil paints or clay, molten silver or a sewing machine, consider how you can play within your current capacity. Honour the minimalism that your circumstance might dictate and see if something emerges with you from your hibernation. Experiment with a child's set of watercolours, squidge play-dough or salt-dough, fiddle with thin and pliable silver wire, collage with glue and fabric scraps. Give yourself time to build on these playthings. Even the work of successful artists can look curiously amateur before completion brings it all together.

Don't be embarrassed to enjoy very simple children's craft kits or art books. I still have a book from when I was 10, that teaches how to draw both cartoon and realistic animals. Embrace whatever fun is within your current abilities. As your health moves into some level of recovery, you may customise and build upon these skills and creations. Perhaps they will be the beginning of a whole new venture? Perhaps not. Just enjoy making use of whatever you can to welcome arts and crafts into your life with minimal stress on your body and mind.

Your health might be preventing you from following your full creative dreams, but an intentional 'let's pretend' project could be the next best thing. Pretend to be what you wish you were. So you can't focus on coherent sentences but you have a vague idea for a book: pretend to be a published author and design your book cover instead. Or build up a series of titles, perhaps even back cover blurbs, in your mind. Just toying freely with ideas may lead to you formulating a more concrete outline that you can develop. Likewise with album covers, if you compose music, or exhibition themes and promotion posters. Visualising a magazine cover that spotlights why they are featuring you in this issue is a fun fantasy project. The artist Grayson Perry did just this, envisioning himself as the rock star he'd like to have been. Designing covers for imaginary fanzines dedicated to his alter ego, he paid homage to a latent aspect of his creative self.

The mini success-story of my magazine (to return to this example for the final time) began when I was emerging from a few years that had seen me often spending over 21 hours a day either asleep or lying down with my eyes shut, sometimes needing assistance to eat or get to the toilet. Tentatively, as I strengthened enough to play with plans again, I toyed with the concept of producing a magazine. I was fortunate in being able to rope in others to assist with typing and other practicalities, but I had no training or expertise. I'd never been well enough to have a job, let alone one in publishing. My exposure to the world of media was only as a consumer. And I was mostly bedbound. But I had nothing to lose. I'd play around from my bed, only doing what I could safely manage without precipitating either a relapse or financial disaster. I'd have fun giving myself the challenge of seeing what transpired. Over time, as my strength reached a slightly higher plateau, the magazine required less input from others and I became its sole editor. The meagre two issues a year didn't seem to me how a proper magazine would operate but it was the most I could offer. They barely earned me any money but that wasn't the point. I broke even and the magazine became my ambassador, with issues looking out on shop floors that I would never visit and speaking to people I wouldn't otherwise have the opportunity to communicate with. My pretending to be a magazine editor resulted in a seven-year life span for *The Triple Spiral* and a great boost to my confidence and creative expression.

If there's something you'd like to do that you can't see how to manifest at your current level of health, ask yourself how you could pretend. You never know where this train of thought may lead but, for now, start with tiny, playful actions.

Cycling on

It can feel an empty, negative, space to be devoid of creative energy, but the path of creativity spirals around. Cycles wrap around in close repetition of earlier ruts and rests while imperceptibly, until you look at the whole picture, moving outwards towards the new. It is not a linear outpouring. There will be times of withdrawing, of questioning, of waiting, and times of expansion, productivity and answers.

I lay for years in the barren, seemingly unharvest-able wasteland of inertia and too-heavy illness. I was always on the lookout, from my pillow, for ways to express my creative self. My attempts, foraged from the undergrowth of fatigue, were occasionally worth saving but I often felt artistically lost. It was one (long) moment in time. More were to come. Different moments, repeating moments, moments of reaping then sleeping. And they all grew from each other: developing, expanding, waiting, achieving, doubting and dreaming. Your time of creation, perhaps in an altered form from the one you've envisaged, will come.

Your time of creation, perhaps in an altered form from the one you've envisaged, will come.

Even if your memory is shot to pieces and your coherence is minimal, everything you've experienced is nestled inside of you, ready to be rejigged and realigned. In time, who knows how much time, it will reappear in a new guise. Don't lose heart. Cast your mind back to what you have enjoyed in the past and trust in the future's potential.

You will have contradictory responses to your situation, many of which you might not feel proud of. These too are all part of the cycle. Acknowledge them without judgement and choose which ones to pay attention to. If darkness weighs you down, consider how it can be used constructively to inform future creations. When inspiration, ability or comfort wanes, rather than pushing murky feelings away, remember the wholeness of the cycle. After all, what is light without shadow in visual art? How can we take sustained pleasure in harmonious notes without pauses or alterations in tempo to offset them? Enforced rest can make the reunion with activity so much more appreciable.

Enforced rest can make the reunion with activity so much more appreciable.

Chapter 18

During a brief return to an art project after a five-year hiatus due to severe ill health, one member of an online craft group, who shares work under the name Soul Treasures, expressed 'feeling very lucky I still have moments that I can be creative. Didn't think it would return any more. Don't know how long it will last but am enjoying every step I can take in the progress of [a *papier maché* lion]. I was almost at a point of discarding it not long ago.' It is so easy to lose motivation or the confidence to continue with creations you have had to set aside. The piece may not yet be looking how you'd imagined and, having not communed with it for a while, you might be doubting the relevance of your vision. Faith in the outcome ebbs and you wonder if half-finished work is just a reminder of what you can no longer do. Like Soul Treasures, we must hold on to our dreams and wait patiently for our body to acquiesce. Reapply yourself when your body and mind concur and see what rekindles. Progress isn't linear. The passing of time, looping back and through repeated cycles, may have generated augmentations to your half-started work.

Don't worry about how slowly your work develops due to the on-again off-again nature of embracing a hobby when chronically ill. All in good time. It is better to go slowly and pay attention to your body setting the pace than to find yourself slipping back into being too unwell to craft at all. Andy, who has severe ME, knows this all too well. Their translation of a haiku by the nineteenth century Japanese poet Issa reminds us of our capabilities if we are compassionate towards our body's need to take things slowly and carefully:

> little snail
> you will climb Mount Fuji
> inch by inch.

If your work in progress is an emotional or expressive piece, your initial desire to express it may have waned. The need to put it out there can become diluted once the bones of the work have been sketched out or scribbled down, causing you to wonder whether it's worth re-engaging with. Sometimes you'll find you've moved on and that's fine. At other times, re-submerging yourself with the original concept may be what's needed to bring your idea to fruition. Remember, too, that it may speak to more people than just yourself.

Fallow time gifts

During the good fortune of better times, it is a powerful act to compassionately prepare for the inevitability of struggle at some point ahead and to make a gift for the future you. Over a few years that consisted of the usual peaks and troughs of chronic illness, I slowly knitted myself that comfort blanket I told you about earlier. When well enough to venture out, I knitted on a lounger in the nearby forest, in bed in a beach hut, or in the garden with the scent of honey from our hive wafting over. When not so well, I knitted with empathy for the pain I was experiencing, patience at not having worked on it for months and alongside the purrs of my elderly cat. My plan was to have memories of what I had managed to enjoy, knowledge that I could withstand difficulties, and self-support knitted into a warm blanket that I could wrap around myself when needed. I ended up benefiting from this sooner than expected as a severe relapse hit out of the blue. The blanket didn't make everything better, but it consoled and held me.

Whichever stage of the cycle you are experiencing, consider how you can prepare for the flipside. Too unwell to create? Perhaps you can browse online for creative books or magazines to gift yourself and feed your inner creator? (Second-hand books and online library resources are great options if money is tight.) Or treat yourself to a handy tool that will make creating easier when you are able to start up again. And if you're currently enjoying creative energy? Gift the future you with some bespoke comfort, be that a cosy blanket, relaxing musical composition, soft teddy, uplifting painting or the creation of a fantasy to escape to in your mind. You are best placed to know what you would most appreciate receiving in your fallow times.

Chapter 18

 Suggested therapeutic activity
Creative comforts

When I was a pre-teen and periodically flattened by symptoms, I made myself a poorly-days entertainment kit. It consisted of a shoebox filled with puzzles and games that I could play with, alone in bed. I would like you to do similar for yourself, focusing on creatively nourishing entertainment for your horizontal days. You may take this literally and fill a container with bed-friendly art and craft supplies, including easy kits that don't require much cognitive effort. You may benefit more from a collection of links to online tutorials, art demonstrations and live story-telling videos; a playlist of easy to consume children's literature, poetry, guided visualisations and relaxing music; a bedside stack of glossy art books, picture books, and anthologies of short writing; or scraps of fabric, tactile pebbles and other textural items to hold and stroke. Arm yourself with a selection of pre-prepared, easy-access creative comforts.

Fallow times and beyond at a glance

- You will have times of inactivity and lack of inspiration, but creative engagement will return.
- Creativity isn't the same as productivity.
- Nurture your dormant self by paying attention to and curating whatever brings you artistic comfort and joy.
- Being an audience to other people's art is a valid involvement with the creative world.
- Cultivate your imaginative skills, even without physically acting on them. Visualise yourself performing your chosen craft.
- Prepare for when you are able to be more active by watching or listening to tutorials and looking at books that bring you a little closer to your goals.
- Jot down any partially formed ideas to refer to when you are able to act on them, or perhaps feel inspired to join these fragments together.
- When energy allows, simply play without expectation of any results.
- When fallow times return, don't despair! Remember that this is part of the natural cycle. You will create again, in one form or another.
- Consider making a gift or survival pack for yourself to benefit from in fallow times.

Part 5:

A dose of inspiration

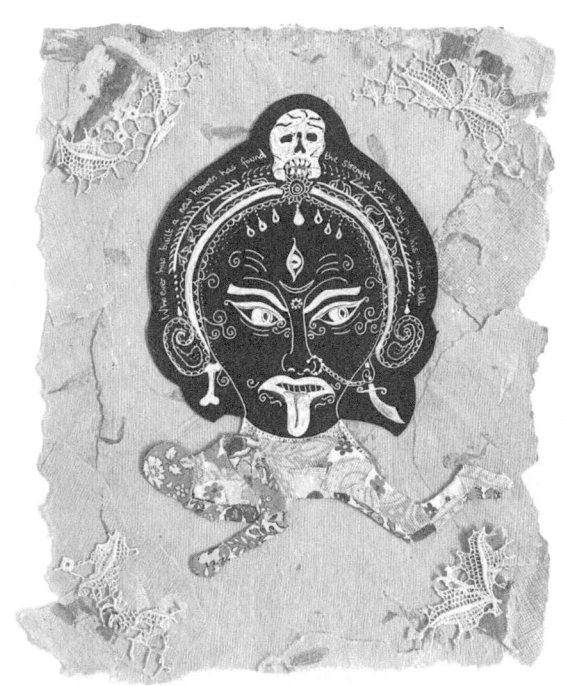

Chapter 19
Changing perception, not circumstance

Writer's block, lack of inspiration and general loss of mojo are familiar to even the healthiest of creatives. Being clinically fatigued, weighed down with pain, frequently confined to the mundanity of home or trapped on a sterile hospital ward are additional factors that can exacerbate inertia. Of course, they may at first trigger a desire to communicate this intense lived experience but, over time, more of the same becomes, well, samey.

Being unwell since childhood, my inner bank of experiences and exposure to different influences has been limited. Art comes from within, but it is fed by stimuli, and we all benefit from new input to shake up our thought processes. On the occasions I could get out to exhibitions or craft shops I would feel a rush of desire to create. My artistic self, when allowed to tentatively explore the big outdoors, would devour the unexpected beauty of layered colour and texture on a rusting object and fatten itself up on the sight of lichened brickwork or an ageing tree trunk. How on earth was I to gather such tasty morsels or maintain motivation when back at home, grounded by illness for vast lengths of time?

Being housebound before the arrival of the internet, I found myself sorely deprived of new input. The feedback and bouncing of ideas to be found within a group of people wasn't available to me and I was lacking in awareness of the various crafts, tools and techniques I could avail myself of. There is no denying that fresh influences do invigorate our creative expression and, thankfully, we now have a multitude of resources just a touchscreen, podcast, or online shop away. Use these to fill yourself with nourishing influences however you are best able and see what happens.

In my inspiration famine, despite my hunger to create, I would question whether I was a naturally creative person if I couldn't summon inspiration wherever I found myself. Would a starving person question whether they are a natural eater because they can't find food within reach? Clearly, that's absurd. But they might need teaching how to catch hidden prey and turn dull looking roots into tasty meals. And that's how it was with me. I needed guidance to learn where the inspiration was hiding.

I gradually learned that being denied access by my condition to activities or places led to an unexpected response. When my mind was given time to come to terms with the lengthy nature of my situation (and it took a long time, I'll be honest) it began to hunt out the interesting and evocative wherever I was. And when I became able to encounter what many others took for granted, I rediscovered a child-like state of wonder. Even experiencing something in a vastly reduced way generated greater awareness of detail and creative motivation than many healthily busy people might experience in a similar situation.

> *My mind began to hunt out the interesting and evocative wherever I was. I rediscovered a child-like state of wonder.*

I remember being well enough to venture out on a mobility scooter one day, not so many years ago, my path taking me on the bridge over a dual carriageway. I felt so high – literally and metaphorically – that I found myself pausing to take a deep breath in awe of this novel experience, waving gleefully at the cars below as they sped beneath me like industrious, colourful ants. I've yet to ever see another adult, without a child in tow, waving at the traffic-ants, and I feel thankful for this perk that my illness bestowed on me.

Similarly, treating ourselves to tiny quantities of food or drink that is usually off limits can enhance our appraisal of textures and flavours and our ability to translate this sensory experience. Just like children responding to all that is new to their world, our imagination can run with the novelty of the rarely visited experience. We can pay attention to our world as though freshly born into it and let our mind play with what it finds. This heightened awareness, un-dampened by familiarity and bursting with detail, can then be moved into our creations.

I now try to embrace this knack that my condition has of encouraging me to experience afresh what others have ceased to appreciate by approaching all encounters, novel or otherwise, with a similar attention. When I can't leave my home, this becomes even more important, reinforced by the novelist Henry Miller's belief that a new environment is never our destination so much as a new perception. Pay attention to objects, textures, sounds and occurrences, even the regular ones in your everyday surroundings, as a new-born or an alien would. Explore them with curiosity and wonder, recognising the detail and raw experience.

And when your health doesn't allow you to either welcome what you've been missing or pay enraptured attention to what is around you, don't worry that you are doing nothing. Change, excitement and focused thought don't always offer the necessary space for the reflection prior to innovation. Creative inspiration likes the still moments and liminal times. When the body is in a safely familiar environment and the mind is given space to just be, inspiration (who is subtle and transient and doesn't like to shout above the hubbub in case it reaches the wrong ears) can make itself heard. It is no coincidence that writers often jump up with an idea just as they are about to fall asleep. This is great news for ill people who are required to be still and restful so much of the time. It has even been asserted that the best ideas arrive when people are tired, due to the less focused brain being more receptive to seeing things in different ways.

Ask your creative self a question and then be patient. Let go but remain open. Harbouring a desperate tension for results will only repel your muse. Sleep on it. Look elsewhere while being alert for her arrival at the edge of your vision.

Encourage yourself to find constructive solutions in unexpected sources. Look to old unfinished projects, meditate on mundanities, form random connections between regular experiences, and welcome familiarity with the curiosity of a newcomer. Let periods of quietude envelop you. Many a poem or creative answer has crept into my awareness while I occupy the relaxed yet attentive space of informal meditation.

> *We don't invent inspiration, we uncover it. And often it is camouflaged right where we are.*

Trying too hard to formulate an original idea is counterproductive. We don't invent inspiration, we uncover it. And often it is camouflaged right where we are. Rather than thinking yourself deeper into the echoes of familiarity, stay exactly where you are but with your mind cocked at a different angle. Like the moment you successfully loosen your gaze when staring at an optical illusion, the hidden image that was in front of you all along may reveal itself. When we mentally scrabble around in search of a forgotten name or word, we use the wrong part of the brain needed for recall and so the memory eludes us. Like the optical illusion, the lost name pops up only when we relax our demand. Inspiration follows the same pattern. Put yourself on standby – receptive and alert – within your same old seemingly unrevealing surroundings. Open the curtains onto your creative self and then, loosening any urgency for a creative vision, metaphorically relax your gaze. Peering over its shoulder repeatedly asking, 'Have you thought of anything yet?' is unlikely to reap rewards.

Used medically, the word inspiration means inhaling. The question then becomes not 'Where can I find inspiration?' but 'What can I creatively inhale from my life and surroundings?' Just as when you breathe your body absorbs oxygen, transfers it to your bloodstream and exhales carbon dioxide, what else can you absorb, transmute and offer back to the world? Inhaling is an automatic action. If we're lucky, we do it with ease. Our conditions may make it feel an effort to suck breath in, or we may need assistance to keep the process flowing smoothly, but if you're reading this then, one way or another, you are breathing. Similarly with creative inspiration. Let it happen. Seek assistance when necessary and be willing to inhale it in an unorthodox way. This may result in crafted output or it may simply entertain your mind as you rest your body. Either is equally valid. Absorb, be mindful, listen, learn, gather, collect and remain receptive to what raises itself for your attention and adaptation. Stay open to the belief that not only does creativity come naturally to you but that inspiration resides wherever you find yourself.

Suggested creative exercises

Welcoming creativity

Look at your immediate environment and, without adding or removing anything, consider how you can perceive it differently. The following suggestions may get you started but the key aim here is to let your own ideas flow, no matter how nonsensical, predictable or wild. Let your creative mind know that it won't be berated for being silly or boring. You are simply giving it space to exercise itself.

- Imagine names and characters for houseplants, trees you can see through the window, ornaments or disability aids.
- Dream up backstories or short magazine articles to accompany any pictures or photographs around you.
- Invent cordon bleu-style names for your everyday meals and snacks.
- Re-name your medication, remedies and therapies as if they are magic spells.
- If the rooms in your home (or wherever you are) were different countries, lands or buildings, what would they be? How would you describe their climate and topography or architecture? What typically happens there? What are the customs and culture?

How many ways?

A popular creative exercise is the thought experiment that asks how many uses you can come up with for a brick. So, how many ways can you think of to use a brick? Don't censor yourself. Explore all possibilities. Outlandish and silly ideas are just as valid as pragmatic, resourceful ones. You are exercising the creative part of your mind, not designing the next best life-hack.

Look around you for other items with which to play this game, or a looser version of it. Ask yourself how regular objects in your environment could be transformed. An old sieve used instead of fabric for cross-stitching, for example. A vintage flour tin as a plant-pot holder. Unworn necklaces or ties used as curtain tiebacks. A spoon bent to become a wall hook. A toothbrush as a broomstick for a mouse-witch. Let your ideas be as practical and implementable or frivolous and fantastical as they like.

Suggested therapeutic activity
Affirming your creativity

Strengthen your awareness of your creative self, even within your restricted experience, with mantras and affirmations such as:
- I am creating a personality to be proud of.
- I am stitching fragments to make something larger than the sum of its parts.
- I notice, appreciate and absorb beauty.
- I am making the most of the life I have.
- I am embellishing my days.
- I am poetry, rap and rhythm.
- I am bled colours and new blends.
- I am colouring in my life.
- I envisage the unseen, the unbeen.
- I am creating.
- I am creation.

Changing perception, not circumstance, at a glance

- A desire to change our circumstances and go seeking inspiration is natural but not necessary.
- Despite potentially monotonous days, inspiration is still hiding all around.
- Pay attention to the mundane in new ways.
- Play differently in your interactions with the world around you.
- Consider how your lifestyle offers you perspectives that many don't spend time with.
- Change your perception around lack of inspiration and let it be, staying alert to creative ideas but without desperation. Invite them to arise without breathing down their neck.

Chapter 20
Moving with the rhythms of restriction

Do you feel as if your illness erects a façade around you, restricting what is seen of your whole self? Do you put a barricade around your illness, trying to hide or transcend it? These limitations on the fullness of you are some of your personal patterns and themes. How can you abstractly, expressively, figuratively or literally depict the rhythm and form of your boundaries and restrictions? How can being attentive to these limitations expose new possibilities and serve you creatively?

When our life has collapsed into stasis and repetition we are given the opportunity to highlight subtle points of interest and the rhythms of restriction. This is where our unique expression lies. Is it possible that what you see as the problem could, in fact, hold the answer? Is it conceivable that your limitations reveal rarely expressed patterns that you can incorporate into your work? Recognising your limitations as a structure that you can work with, instead of an untouchable barricade, is where creativity emerges.

Does your enforced sedentary lifestyle allow you to gently stitch away, at your own pace, in a way that a healthy version of you might never have explored? Can your limitations, then, be used to frame a focused outlook, metaphorically or more literally? Perhaps, in some fashion, they build a safe harbour to contain the more accessible rhythms of an ocean of opportunities?

Sometimes total freedom is more inhibiting than having to work within boundaries. Too much choice can make us freeze, opt for the status quo, or endlessly vacillate; too much time and we procrastinate and postpone. In a restrictive situation, however, we are guided as to where to turn our attention. Being ill is a monotonous business – one that leaves us wishing for the freedom to choose from the possibilities, beyond the safe harbour, on the sea's horizon – but it needn't cut us off completely from our creativity. It can hone our interests and the rhythms our creativity dances to. We can still feel the edge of the ocean wash through us, ripple over us, delivering its patterns in the sand.

And yet, still, an atmosphere of stagnation can accompany chronic illness. Days and nights are as fixed as possible to the routine that serves our body. Stuck in one building or room, stuck in our ailment, stuck in a life that doesn't deliver the pathways we expected for ourselves, we can feel bereft of spontaneous movement. How do we get things moving when both our body and creativity feel trapped by restrictions?

Patterns and designs are comprised of restriction and repetition.

First, recognise that patterns and designs are comprised of restriction and repetition. Musical rhythms consist of a select use of sounds and rests, phrased and repeated by the composer. Even the more exuberant movements of experimental dance, while welcoming diversity, stick to a relatively structured pattern in time with the music. It's true that music consisting of one long static note isn't music at all, and your life may feel like a droning singular tone, but listen carefully. There will be vibrations and minute variations in the steady hum of your existence. You can build on these.

The re-run of relapses and strobe-lit pain, that self-preservation insists I partially forget, periodically pinpricks any complacent comfort, creating repeat channels for new self-expression to leak out. And then, after the depths, the child-like delight at regaining a simple ability, such as standing in rain outside the back door, sparks a desire to share the intensity of the moment. In these ways, with these patterns, existence rocks a vibrant rhythm to explore.

Chapter 20

Remind yourself that things are always changing and moving at some level. The shadows in the room travel with the day, seasons turn, cobwebs increase or are cleared away, the floor accumulates patterns of dirt, symptoms migrate, pain levels fluctuate, emotions flatten and heighten. We can turn our attention to the minutiae of the vastness within and around us, rather than the seemingly solid axis of our illness around which the world turns. Look for what has changed or is moving within your experience and see if it sparks a desire to explore or depict it. Watch the flights and behavioural patterns of birds and insects. Weather watch, neighbourhood-cat watch, moon watch, leaf watch. Open a window or door and feel the wind on your skin. These observations and sensations can shift you beyond the tethers of confinement and into new perceptions, without requiring you to be anywhere other than where you are.

By becoming attentive to the ever-moving ride that is the daily, weekly, seasonal or less predictable rhythms of life, we might recognise secure foundational patterns and recurring motifs, as well as the contrast of raised relief that we prefer to encounter. What we had taken to be a bland straight line of merely coping, it turns out, has gullies and peaks and shade and light; depth enough to work with.

There is no denying that novel experiences with the natural world are one of the strongest influences on my creativity. Being so limited in how far I can travel or move around within the wider landscape is, therefore, undoubtedly a hindrance. But, as well as the open doorway of the internet, there are other ways of welcoming the new into my restricted life and thus turning what could be interpreted as a motionless existence into a more rhythmically inspiring one.

We can unite ourselves with the movement of the outer world by creatively honouring the recurrences of the turning year. Limited in the places and social events we can attend, we learn to pay attention to the rhythmic events and rituals we do have access to. The turning seasons reach into my bedroom through the window, each repetition feeling simultaneously nostalgic and new. Spring and summer see my writing more influenced by the natural world as open windows usher in the outside, and lying on the ground outdoors becomes possible. Autumn encourages me to welcome the act of hunkering down, preparing for the chill with knitting and patchwork. Christmas is rapidly followed by my birthday and these two events so close together, if I'm lucky, supply a selection of books and art or craft equipment, triggering different approaches and renewed motivation or vicarious involvement. Rhythm, movement, connection and novelty are available to me, without immersion in what is currently unreachable.

Whether you choose religious celebrations, the more nature-based festivals of the Celtic wheel of the year or your own annual marker points, through observing the movement of the year you access the many changes and patterns happening around you. In this way you both expand your personal rhythms to encompass the wider world and you contract nature until it fits your experience. As John Fox, the author of *Poetic Medicine*, has observed, the personal and the universal become reflections of each other. Through exploring this, we can accept the movement of our inner experiences as natural and discover relatable ways of expressing them creatively, as well as reconnecting ourselves with the world outside.

> *Through observing the movement of the year you access the rhythms around you.*

All forms of creativity have the power to re-connect us with the world we had begun to feel separate from, helping us respond to the wider movements of the world, metaphorically or explicitly exploring motion and harnessing action. Art historian and psychologist Tobi Zausner notes how Toulouse-Lautrec compensated for not being able to ride the horses he loved (probably due to pycnodysostosis, a rare genetic condition also known as Toulouse-Lautrec syndrome) by frequently painting them so that he could sense the rhythmic leap of the horse for the time in which he was painting it, freeing himself temporarily from his physical confines.

Chapter 20

The stab of needle and flow of thread when sewing is another way of replacing interminable stillness with both cathartic and pleasing movement. Just as Toulouse-Lautrec found with the subject matter of his paintings, it is enhanced further when combined with depictions of lost experiences. In her fascinating book *Threads of Life*, Clare Hunter describes how, in the aftermath of a brain abscess that left a fisherman increasingly ill, he first took to painting oil and watercolour seascapes, and making toy boats, and then, as his health confined him more and more to his bed, discovered embroidery. Using scraps of fabric and basic stitches taught to him by his wife, he learnt to depict the movement of sand dunes and waves. As threads instead of sand spilled through his hands, and the needle moved up and down, he returned in his memory to the seaside and the rock and the swell of the ocean.

Using various aspects of creativity, we can embrace both the energising and the soothingly familiar patterns that roll on by while we abide in our limited crease of the universe. I have known chronically ill photographers who are too unwell to leave their beds, focus their eyes, hold their arms steady or let much light into their space – conditions which many would assume preclude them from their art – capture appealing and thought-provoking pictures. Taking photographs of shadow lives and rays of light that creep around curtains can be surprisingly powerful. Moving the camera as a shot is taken can result in stylistically blurred images, streaks of light, and unexpected images artistically emphasising one's experience of unsteadiness and the speed of life moving around one's prone form. These can be satisfying images as they are, or translated into other media.

No matter how much movement we aim to portray in our work, the sloweddown, stuck-in-the-mud reality of living with chronic illness is an inhibiting factor for those who gain inspiration while physically on the move. For them, the metaphor of beautiful lotus flowers blooming in mud is of no comfort. 'Composing on the lips' is a method for freeing up stuck creativity by speaking ideas into a voice note or Dictaphone while walking. The experience for many is that having their senses engaged in physical movement and changing scenery releases them from a creative block. How can we achieve a similar effect when our ability to walk, or indeed move much at all, may be restricted?

If you can go for a wheelie-walk using a wheelchair or mobility scooter, or be taken on a short drive, these will provide an awareness of movement and change, no matter that your limbs aren't active. It is interesting to note, after long periods of being housebound, how strongly one's body responds to being in a moving vehicle. These are sensations perhaps never noticed by healthier travellers but available to the artist in you. Perhaps you can manage a miniature walk into your garden or just down the front path and back, absorbing the change of perspective and any differences from last time you were able to stand there. The fact that such activities can exhaust us demonstrates the sensory input involved and the contrast between these activities and our resting life, implying that we can utilise even the tiniest of excursions.

Without moving elsewhere at all, tai chi, yoga, a few stretches, or even gentler movements such as deep breathing or tensing and relaxing muscles, can allow the conscious mind's grip to loosen a little, leading us not into new vistas but perhaps into new recognitions of experience. Similarly, using our senses to appreciate external movements can help us to draw upon the patterns and rhythms of motion. Feeling individual and collective drops of shower water hitting your shoulders and running down your back; sloshing your hands or feet in a bowl of water; making waves in the bath; listening to a small battery-operated water feature or delicate wind chimes; having a massage or somebody gently stroking your head – these are all ways to absorb the impression of movement in a generally stationary situation. Embraced with full attention, they offer the possibility of shifting us out of a stultified mindset and into an active, albeit restricted, experience, perhaps enabling us to add extra dimensions to our creative pursuits.

Suggested creative exercise
Repeating patterns

Experiment with designing repeating patterns inspired by your personal restrictions. You might choose to investigate the way your illness limits your life in general or focus on a particular aspect of your experience. Consider how straight lines, curves, harsh marks, soft shading, textures, sounds, shapes, colours, materials and stitches can be employed to represent various aspects of the rhythm you are confined to. Your rhythm may not be smooth or regular. In capturing it artistically you might discover more variation in your life than you had previously realised. It just happens to be a different rhythm from the one you might have wanted.

Suggested therapeutic activities
(Internal) weather

Knit, crochet, weave or patchwork a blanket or scarf that records either the literal weather or your predominant symptoms and/or emotions, allocating a different colour to each condition you are likely to experience and adding a couple of rows or patches every day. Using two or three strands of yarn at once, multicoloured fabric or visible sewing, you can highlight a few prominent features from each day. Other media, from colouring, cross-stitch or paper collages to beadwork, mosaics or painting also lend themselves to themed projects that chart weather, air temperature, symptoms or emotions.

You may, instead, choose to record the highest/lowest daily air temperature, intensity/relief of one key symptom, or any other regular variations – whatever best reflects, for you, the pattern of your days.

If symptoms prevent you working daily, make a brief note of each day's weather so that you can catch up when feeling up to it. At the end of a year, you will have a colourful record of the internal or seasonal pattern of your year, regardless of how limited you may have felt the outward expression of your life to be at the time. While creating this artistic response to quotidian observations, you may (or may not – which can be a revelation in itself) become more aware of interlinked patterns emerging between different aspects of your life.

For more ideas around this, look online for guidelines on creating temperature blankets and temperature art.

Restriction wall

Depict, in the medium of your choice, a restriction wall. Do all the bricks represent the same restrictions bearing down on you or is each one different? Does a pattern emerge? Do you want to create a piece of art featuring just one of the bricks in the wall? Is it not a wall at all, but a hedge or fence or something else entirely? Are your restrictions dense and unyielding or flexible with gaps in between? Can you find a rhythm of any relief or mitigation running through this wall? What is this division constructed from – other people's comments blocking you from intimacy or understanding; limited access to medical care; symptoms causing you to miss out on things; inaccessibility preventing you from attending social places; emotions around accepting your illness? Does this wall, or at least some of the components of it, protect or serve you in any way? Can you turn these restrictions or this art piece into a positive perspective or is it simply cathartic? Perhaps it could be shared online to raise awareness.

Moving with the rhythms of restriction at a glance

- Even when your life feels motionless there are rhythms to be creatively mined.
- Restrictions that feel all-encompassing have their own rhythms to be explored.
- Rhythms of the natural world and the turning year may be accessible inspiration.
- Rhythms of your body and mind can influence your art.
- Consider how you could recreate in your work the rhythmic movements of activities you used to, or would now like to, engage in.
- Invite movement into your life in whatever way you can – through any of your senses, and only as much as is comfortable – to awaken new creative responses.

Chapter 21
Going without

Here, we follow on from the theme of restriction but, rather than studying the patterns we can recognise in our limitations, we embrace what is missing and look for the creative benefits of going without something. I often get carried away with how many gorgeous influences could be included in a piece of work but am learning that a reduced colour palette or more focused theme can benefit the outcome. In both art and life, it can be what you leave out, as much as what you keep in, that has the best effect.

Ahmet Altan, a writer and journalist incarcerated under political charges in a Turkish prison cell, wrote about the sparsity of prison life fuelling his creativity. Even his words had to be creatively smuggled out in order to be shared with the world. Goodness knows, severe long-term ill health can feel like a life sentence, imprisoned as we are behind the barbed-wire pain and concrete restrictions of our conditions. Denied quick fixes and easy pleasures, like Altan we learn to be resourceful. We can loosen our grip on what we wish we had in favour of considering what can be made with what we do have. Unable to mooch around shops for materials, or galleries for inspiration, we are forced, if we want to feel fulfilled, to recognise the uses of what may otherwise have been dismissed or gone unnoticed. We develop more original creative pathways.

Yes, we can purchase most of what we desire at the click of a button now, but I'm impatient. When I feel the delicious combination of both an idea and the energy to give it a go I don't want to wait for a delivery before I can get started. I also derive greater pleasure from recycling what is around me and transforming the unused. Therefore, when I don't have the desired colour, yarn or fabric, I use whatever I can lay my hands on to colour what I do have while my body is feeling amenable. Tea, coffee, turmeric, beetroot and watered-down fabric paint have all been applied to textiles in my kitchen. A left-over tin of white emulsion paint has served me well for block printing. The creative cooks and bakers among you will know the frustration of not having a key ingredient to hand. In times of lack, don't give up: substitute. Experiment and discover new flavour-buddies. It is said that recipes such as Waldorf salad, Bakewell tart and Vichyssoise all came into being due to a lack of other ingredients.

Limited resources encourage ingenuity and resourcefulness. This window of energy, this restricted movement, this store of materials and household items, is all we have so let's work with it while we can and see what emerges. But going without needn't just be an enforced situation. It can be an adaptive and creative skill that we consciously practise. An important part of the creative process is recognising when to set aside some of what you'd like to include because it is muddying the message or scattering attention. Know when to stop!

Going without is an adaptive and creative skill that we can consciously practise.

In a similar way, limited craft sessions can be regarded as a consciously imposed positive force rather than merely curtailing our fun. Less is more, says our body, and we can choose to agree. The restrained timeframe focuses our attention towards achieving the maximum we can within that boundary. Knowing that if I procrastinate I won't have anything to see for my small window of activity, I am spurred on to spill whatever ideas or abilities may be residing in me. This isn't about rushing but about honing my instincts to recognise what feels most relevant. Even when inspiration is thin, I am encouraged to do something – anything – with this allocated time. And when time runs out on this session, rather than feeling the frustration of downing tools, we can consider this an opportunity for our still ticking creativity to edit and mould what we have begun, without the pressure of action or the risk of hasty moves. The pathway for inspiration has been opened; now we watch to see what arrives. Structured time-out can be considered the white space of our creative time, giving the mind an uncluttered arena to process and respond to the work in progress.

In design, white space refers to the empty space on the page, completely unoccupied by text or images. The more professional the designer, the more white space is paid attention to and employed. Similarly, negative space is a term that describes the empty shapes between solid objects. In traditional Japanese arts and culture, negative space is called *ma*. The attention paid to *ma* is often considered as important as any other aspect of a piece of artwork for drawing the viewer's eye and creating effect. We can embrace this concept by taking interest in the spaces alongside that which we would ordinarily notice. What is revealed by going without certain objects or abilities? What inspiration resides in absence and shortage? Rather than bemoaning a lack of bounteous resources, health-wise or otherwise, be curious about what you are left with.

When devoid of ideas, or confused into stasis by too many possibilities, I have found it beneficial to give myself a deliberate limitation to work with. At first frustrating, this chosen omission provides a welcome structure. Deliberately denying yourself something might feel perverse when you already experience so much restriction, but it can be surprisingly empowering. Actively choosing something extra to go without lends a sense of control when you might otherwise feel powerless or directionless. Denial guides us down potentially rewarding avenues we might otherwise never have explored. In the face of a deliberate restriction, I look for unusual alternatives and edit myself to unexpectedly positive ends.

Conversely, perhaps self-censorship is the thing you could experiment with forsaking. Drawing or writing in ink instead of pencil so that you are forced to go without the luxury of erasing any mistakes has, at times, resulted in surprisingly better results for me. I have been obliged to stay with what I didn't like and build upon it, incorporating or transforming it and making creative breakthroughs rather than shying away due to lack of instant ability.

If inspiration is still not forthcoming, rather than trying to force ideas, accept that novelty may not be on the agenda now. Forget about it. Forego innovation for a while, consolidating past practice and designs instead. Settle with the familiar and wait this time out. You may find that focusing on a tried-and-tested speciality is where you choose to stay. Take comfort in what you do have at your disposal, without taxing your limited resources, and recognise an apparently empty mind as a receptive and welcoming area.

Having realised the importance of sparsity, relax into the space that is left by it. Acknowledged for what it is – a pause between activities, ability, or inspiration – it becomes less frightening. It isn't all encompassing or eternal and is thus less overwhelming to experience than you had feared. Stay without for a while. Take a rest. Welcome a different perspective by being on the outside looking in.

Some of you may be shouting 'But it's not just a pause "between"; those opportunities are gone from me for good!' and I hear you. Coming to terms with what we have lost or may never have had is hard – really hard. It's also surprising how we find new routes towards pleasure and creativity. Accepting that you can't do what you'd like isn't resignation. It doesn't mean you've reconciled yourself with going without forever. It is an adjustment. You and your body can work together to find alternative ways of expressing your creativity.

Lean into this absence of what you'd love to embrace and allow echoes of it to be present in your reconsidered creativity. This is one way of maintaining a connection with what feels snatched from your lived days. I once heard of a diabetic baker who couldn't eat any of her cakes but loved to make them for friends and family. Her inability to consume home-cooked sweetness hadn't robbed her of her joy in baking cakes.

Chapter 21

I often feel that others must assume the limited life I live is a reflection of my personality as much as being foisted on me by illness. Just like the cake-lover who doesn't eat them, my body mis-portrays me as a sedately sensible creature of caution. But just because I'm never seen dancing, hiking, wild swimming or night gallivanting doesn't mean that's not what I get up to in my dreams. To overcome this, I have begun to create art that highlights the dissonance between what I'm forced to go without and what my spirit yearns for. I have learned that creatively expressing what resides in the apparent emptiness also connects me with others. By expressing what you thought was uniquely visceral to you, you become a representative for that which may have gone without recognition or open acknowledgment.

> *I have begun to create art that highlights the dissonance between what I'm forced to go without and what my spirit yearns for.*

Suggested creative exercises

Attention to negative space

Create a piece of art that relies on negative space to define what is around it. Your artistic skill isn't important. This exercise is to encourage recognition of the value of gaps in their own right, without distorting what is around that empty space. Begin by drawing or painting a picture not by focusing on any solid objects but by depicting the spaces between them. A simple way into this technique is to look at a slatted chair back, a bare-branched tree or an enlarged photo of a snowflake and draw only the gaps. Observe the spaces between what is there so attentively that when you draw the emptiness you reveal a picture of the object. This is harder than it sounds!

If drawing isn't your thing, move on to your chosen craft to examine negative space. Write about something without mentioning it specifically, obliquely referencing it through what skirts around it and defines its presence. Knit in lace stitch or use textiles in other ways that rely on the unoccupied places and empty gaps to create the pattern. Create music that relies on quiet rests. Sculpt a bowl or other object that is formed around hollow space.

Self-denial

Deny yourself something you'd normally use in your art – a particular colour, stitch, letter of the alphabet, punctuation mark or creative tool. Contain yourself artificially with a limited palette, highly structured poetic form, specific word count, or no paintbrush and see what exists beyond the omission of freedom.

Suggested therapeutic activity
Would if I could

Produce a creation that demonstrates something your health forces you to live without. This isn't an exercise in self-pity or adding salt to the wound. Use this project as an opportunity to celebrate what you would love to embrace, to share aspects of your personality that don't get a chance to shine, or to work through anger and disappointment. My 'Would if I Could' collage, made from hand-torn and stitched maps surrounding a paper-cut silhouette of my head containing destinations I would love to travel to, is pictured at the beginning of Part 6 of this book.

Going without at a glance

- Going without something can influence our creativity in ways we may not have explored given freedom of choice.
- Aesthetically, less is often more.
- Creativity often stems from a desire to resolve a problem. How can what you are having to go without inspire creative direction?
- Having limited available energy can encourage us to make the most of moments of activity. This can be seen as a motivational gift rather than a curse.
- Consider the concepts of white space and negative space. These gaps on the page, between physical objects, or in life itself, are just as important as what is consciously noticed.
- For now, pay less attention to the obvious and hone your awareness to the apparent gaps and emptiness, and what quietly dwells therein.
- It may seem perverse, but giving yourself extra limitations can enhance your creativity. Consider reducing your colour palette, word count, or what you include in a composition.
- Consider how your creations can represent what you are forced to go without, integrating these losses back into your life in some form or another.

Chapter 22
Going within

Inside you, behind the multi-storey tower blocks of ailments and pain, beyond the wastelands of fatigue, are exquisite shores of possibility. This is where hopes and plans come from afar to drop anchor. Some stay while others take off again to gather more curios. Flotsam and jetsam reveal themselves to be not litter but treasures and fragments for upcycling. This is where you can go to replenish your spirit, creative or otherwise. If you haven't yet discovered this place within, trust that it exists and embark on an inner exploration.

Close your eyes and visualise the pathway. At first it may reveal tombstones to the past, or megaliths in your way. It is entirely up to you whether you sit with these for a while, seeing what they have to offer, or move straight past. What comes into view? Vistas recalled from film scenes, dream destinations, memories of places visited? Is this creative repository inside of you open and expansive or do you find yourself inside a museum of curiosities, a cave of smuggled inspiration, a maze of opportunities and dead ends? Are there detailed images, deeply carved sentences, amorphous colour-shrouded feelings?

When your body limits your outer world adventures your inner world becomes paramount. Indeed, the poet Rainer Maria Rilke argued that the only true journey is the one each of us takes inside of ourselves. Some people disappear easily into detailed fantasies, using them to immerse themselves in comfort, respite and imaginative concepts. Others, and I fall into this category, find mental visualisations tricky to pin down and tiring to focus on. I don't form pictures in my mind easily but when I employ words the images begin to write themselves.

Shortcuts to help you onto a more scenic inner path include guided visualisations, music, sounds of nature or evocative scents. I can often be found indulging in a deep sniff of some forbidden food being eaten near me. I take my time to focus on ingesting the fragrance and visualising the particles of pleasure travelling into me. As I consume the treat in my own way, I summon the sensory experience I crave. Experiment with different stimuli to find the pathway your brain best uses to carry you on an inward journey.

Of course, one of our richest inner hoards is our bank of memories, ripe for creative adaptation. Reminiscing brings the past into contact with the present, carrying the potential to trigger a creative avenue that hadn't made itself obvious before. When the present is dreary or difficult, aspects of the past may be a comforting refuge. Can far-off memories decorate your present thoughts, supplying material for you to patchwork and fold, repeat-print and hold – metaphorically or otherwise? Use any evocative shortcuts (fragrance, music, taste, texture, photographs…) to open the doorway directly onto these memories. Then explore and play with them. Re-work them, if necessary, in a way that informs your creativity and expands your current situation.

> *Far-off memories can decorate your present thoughts, supplying material for you to patchwork and fold, repeat-print and hold – metaphorically or otherwise.*

The destination of your inner journey will be richer to draw from if the inside of your mind is already a widely sourced collage. If you haven't had the opportunity to build a preparatory bank of inspirational memories or influences, it is never too late to start. In the fragility of your current situation, you may feel too unwell to entertain diverse images and influences but perhaps you can let soothing colours and simple sensations wash over and through you. Different textures, picture books, gently descriptive audiobooks, lilting music. You may manage spoken radio or podcasts bringing information that you can silence at will, or slow TV featuring real-time canal boat or train journeys. Absorb what you can when you can.

Chapter 22

Be aware that journeying inwards isn't all summoned scenes and bright memories, and that this is right and normal. When symptoms and events are especially hard, the recesses and crevices of your being offer refuge to all the (metaphorical) demons attracted to darkness. I won't tell you not to be afraid. Deep monochrome looms amorphously, layer upon layer of more greys and blacks than you knew possible. Fear is natural (and some chronic illness symptoms emulate the physical effects of it all by themselves). I will, however, ask you to remember that you are far stronger, more multi-dimensional and longer living, than any of those dark spectres. Dare to probe these shades of darkness, the umbral and penumbral areas where light struggles to reach. What phantoms and fungi, lichens and ghosts reside here? They are opportunistic but you are investigative. You know that not only is there light beyond them that they are reluctant to turn to but that you can sap their power by filtering it into your art. Mourn. Be honest. Be dark and muddy and loud and courageous and raggedy and blurred and demonstrative in your suffering. Give yourself permission to really feel what has been side-lined as negative while you transmute these uncomfortably ignored tones, textures and words and redeem them as art.

Perhaps you can consider the subterranean travels that illness sends you on not as hijackings but merely the more perilous stages of your creative adventure from which you will one day return, carrying with you story- or picture-prompting artefacts. The closer you can observe your inner terrain the more you bring back to deliver to your creations when the energy takes you. What you choose to create may be visibly representative of your inner experience or it may reveal nothing of its origins to the viewer. A hand-knitted black bouclé beanie hat or a fantasy tale may be the result of your inner journey, with only you aware of how your situation informed its conception or of how cathartic the creation process proved to be.

The closer you can observe your inner terrain, the more you bring to your creations when the energy takes you.

Put your responses to the difficulties life presents you with into your art rather than letting them roam gloomily through your life. The last thing you want is them skulking, ominously unrecognised, in your personality's hidden corners when they could be transformed into something breath-taking, awareness-making, liberating.

You may have developed some eccentric perspectives, unusual coping mechanisms or found that your soul is lifted with distinctive colours or wild desires, thanks to your experiences. Claim these quirks and use them. Rather than wishing you could fit in or be more 'normal', own your originality and what sets you apart as interesting. Listening to an interview with author Alice Sebold some fifteen years ago changed my attitude to myself from that day onwards. She talked about feeling different from others but learning to inhabit what she perceived as her weirdness, and I have endeavoured to do exactly this ever since.

Going within is also how we better respond to what is around us. By synchronising our outer awareness with our inner journey we travel deeper into what we are seeing, hearing, feeling or remembering. Pay attention to the fullness of all your senses, rather than relying on what hearsay, habit or cursory attention assumes is there. And if your senses distort reality – well, there is a new perception ripe for portrayal. Art is about combining the essence of what you are depicting with your own experience and personality.

Embrace aspects of yourself and your creativity that you may have previously dismissed, attempted to erase or pushed shamefully under the carpet. Go into them and see where they may take you. No matter if they turn out to be dead ends – one of them may be a cul-de-sac with a surprising internal view.

Suggested creative exercise
Follow the scent

Choose a fragrance you can tolerate – if not a perfume, essential oil or incense, then a fragrant leaf, flower, spice jar, slice of citrus fruit, cup of smoky Lapsang

Souchong tea, or an open window – and sit or lie down with it near you. Close your eyes – perhaps wear a sleep mask and ear plugs to focus entirely on your sense of smell – and follow the scent as it travels up your nostrils and into your olfactory system. What does this smell evoke for you? Memories, feelings, desires? Colours, tactile sensations, warmth, cold? How would you describe the scent and where does it take you? If it had a voice, what would it say? Use this exercise to sharpen your awareness of inner experiences and how they combine with external stimuli to spark creative thoughts.

Suggested therapeutic activities
Self-portrait

This self-portrait might look nothing like your physical self, and it needn't be a drawing or painting. Be it sketch, poem, sculpture, clothing, music, creature, puddle of colours, or whatever comes to mind, aim to represent your inner self. This could be a general depiction of who you feel yourself to be on the inside or one aspect that you want to focus on. Consider the following questions before starting your piece:

- Do you want to express your core values or passions?
- Would you like to draw out dark emotions?
- Do you want to re-discover personal joy that has been buried deep?
- Could you benefit from addressing how your self-image has changed with the progression (or stagnation) of your illness?
- How do you see yourself? Is this how you want others to see you or are these two very different images?
- Is there a concealed or misunderstood aspect of yourself that you would like to share in the safe space of your portrait?
- Does depicting your inner self make you want to work quickly, carefully, freely, abstractly, intricately, methodically…? What does this say about your relationship with yourself and how you can become more constructively in touch with your inner experiences?
- Will you keep this portrait? Will you share it?

Inner amulet

An amulet is a symbolic object or image used to invoke protection or positive outcome. It might be a piece of jewellery; a design applied to clothing; a mojo pouch containing a written charm along with herbs, crystals and animal representations; or any other talismanic keepsake. The colours, images and materials are chosen with care to bestow the desired effect. Although often beautiful, it is intent and personal meaning, rather than aesthetic talent, that are primarily poured into the making of talismans.

If able, research traditional talismanic designs from various cultures as well as considering the qualities that different creatures, people, plants, colours, patterns, shapes and materials evoke for you. Then design and make (if you wish – this can be a thought creation as much as a physical one) an amulet to enhance your sense of comfort, support and personal power.

Your amulet may be as simple as an origami heart or a two-line chant. It may be a hand-sewn doll, small enough to sit in the palm of your hand, or a Native American-inspired medicine shield. Is it an embodiment of your inner strength, to remind you that you can rely on yourself to cope with hard times, or does it contain elements from the wider world for when life inside your body and mind requires outside assistance? Have fun taking time to connect constructively with your inner self.

Going within at a glance

- Take a journey inside yourself and see what you find along the way.
- You may discover joyful memories, fantasy visions or hungry ghosts – these can all be integrated into your creativity.
- Guided visualisations, photographs from your past, and evocative scents, tastes and sounds can all help you travel deeper within.
- The more your inner landscape is fed, the vaster it grows. Fatten it up by absorbing facts, nature photographs and fantasy images.
- Instead of making assumptions about what you are experiencing, pay attention to all of your senses and how they are processing and interpreting the world around you.
- Own your oddities, capitalise on your quirks, and investigate previously rejected aspects of yourself. These are what will bring extra depth to your work.

Chapter 23
Listening to the voice of illness

The classic advice to authors is to write what you know, and what do we know better than the tumult of our own body's experience? Even if you see arts and crafts as escapism from illness, incorporating the unique voice of your own ill body can lend originality to your work.

The voice of illness is sometimes sledgehammer direct, brutal and to the point. At other times it is more surreal, abstract, or impressionistic – a delayed echo at the edges of understanding. Be curious about the variability and specificity of bodily sensations, willing to listen with interest. This isn't easy when we, naturally, don't want to hear what is being conveyed. One way to work with this resistance is to translate a language you find particularly ugly or frightening into one you can more easily sit with. When listening creatively to the language of our body, this means switching senses and seeing how else we can interpret its collection of messages.

Just as someone with synaesthesia may naturally attribute colours to sounds, are you more able to respond to your symptoms by translating them into another sense? What colour, texture, shape, density or sound does a particular pain, restriction or discomfort embody? Is it static, pulsing, undulating? Does it stay put or roam around in space, time and between senses? Does it have distinct or blurred boundaries? Re-structuring your awareness of symptoms in this way can enable a more objective and less habitual or fearful relationship with your body, as well as inspiring novel interpretations to include in your body of work.

> *Be willing to listen with interest to the language of your body.*

Extricating yourself from a shared identity with your symptoms can be tricky. Our body is our only contact with the physicality of the world, so it is understandable when we lose objectivity and become submerged in visceral sensations. To help step outside of ourselves and gain a fresh perspective we can ask ourselves how a poet, a sculptor, a painter, a musician might represent our current suffering. Given this doorway into a different viewpoint, our mind may surprise us with powerful images that can serve us both emotionally and creatively.

Hyper-sensitivity lends itself particularly to this approach. It's hard to be with the screeching cacophony your senses present you with when they've lost their filter. Your brain is bombarded with nauseatingly flickering movement or has its volume ramped up, sometimes indiscriminately, sometimes on one persistent electrical hum or beep (the stairlift across the landing from my bedroom, in my case), sometimes on the bellowing assault of tinnitus. Here, again, it can be therapeutic to just stay with this sensation, inquisitively paying attention to the patterns, movements, colours and obliterations within. Rather than trying to ignore this barrage or push through it to focus on what you were trying to do, give it your attention, just for as long as you can bear. See if you discover anything of interest to bring back from this experience and deliver into your work.

It has been said that Proust's attention to detail in his writing is a side effect of his body's hyper-sensitivity to his surroundings. When textures of clothing become augmented on skin, light feels like harsh metal spoons curving behind eyeballs to scoop them out, and movement in peripheral vision sends the body onto a storm-tossed ship we are invited, if we wish, to make something from these visceral components. As well as instigating artistic self-expression or an increased awareness of the power of texture in your made objects, honing your awareness of your senses and cross-referencing these experiences creates powerful imagery. This in turn provides a way to externalise internal discomfort and represent symptoms that others may not readily understand.

Your health can also lend its voice to your art when it creates adaptive pathways that result in original effects. Aphasia, or difficulty with word recall, is a prime example. Mahli appealed in an online group for other people's brain fog induced 'funny descriptors'. From the likes of 'fuel teapot' (petrol pump), 'cowlet' (calf), 'long-necked horse' (giraffe) and 'baby Jesus pizza' (mince pie) she created an illustration called Brain Fog Brainwaves. If you like writing surreal fiction, then consider casting brain fog as your collaborator. My brain, once using the word 'trousers' instead of traffic, instigated a fun session drawing a cartoon that the intended sentence would never have led to.

Getting creative with the raw materials of lived illness leads me to think of trench artists in the first and second world wars. Trench art was the name given to arts and crafts made by soldiers as rehabilitation therapy as well as by civilians from the materials left lying around in the aftermath of conflict. Without having to perceive your condition as a battle you might still embrace the idea of being a trench artist, utilising not just the sensations and events but also the cast-offs of your situation.

Medicine bottles, boxes and tablet blister sheets, compression stockings, inhaler components, quotes from health care workers, and other by-products of living with illness may all find a home in your work – the debris of illness becoming the voice of expression. In this way, your materials can do some of the work for you before you even begin. Using bandages or a well-worn nightshirt in textile art, or old prescription slips in papercraft, starts the story before we bring structure and embellishments along to lead us deeper. When we do add our own touches, we can think how the next layer of materials converses with the primary message. Charcoal, considering how it was born from burning wood, lends itself to communicating transformation. Its colour and the imprecise marks it is so good at making also impart pure, unrefined expression of dark emotions. Watercolours intimate gentleness or the flow of emotion. Pens tend to denote articulacy, definition and permanence. Whether words or colours are your chosen media, select them with this same attention to what they instinctively convey, as well as considering how you can lift them from familiar usage into strategic arrangements that vocalise your intent.

Having focused primarily on the heavier aspects of all that illness may want to voice, let's conclude this chapter by remembering that the voice of illness is multifaceted. It doesn't just obsess over a litany of symptoms and medical treatments or cathartic processes. Illness knows the value of compassion and, as such, you may detect it encouraging you to make comforting and uplifting items for yourself and others. It asks for self-care and distraction through comfort, humour, little luxuries and elements of nature. Listen to these requests, too, and turn your creativity towards whatever you hear a desire for.

Illness asks for self-care, comfort, humour, little luxuries and elements of nature.

Suggested creative exercises
A conversation with pain (or discomfort)

With your eyes shut and resting in as comfortable a position as possible, imagine you are an artist or crafter in any genre you desire. This needn't be one that you have any talent for or accessibility to, just one that grabs your fancy for this exercise. In your chosen role, objectively interview a symptom that you are currently experiencing. Ask it how it would like you to depict it in the medium of this craft. Observe it while discussing how you envisage representing its raw state and see what new perceptions, acceptance, understandings or ideas may arise.

Can your inner observational artist sit with this unpleasant symptom and notice fluctuations, interesting sensations or previously unexplored aspects of it that will help you to experience it more creatively? Play with translating your mindful experience into colours, textures and shapes, sequences, motifs or stand-alone imagery. Perhaps you can imagine the symptom as an animal or quirky character residing inside you, going about their personal business or duties. Directing your attention in this way is helpful both as an instigator to artistic responses and as a creative coping technique when pain or discomfort are taking centre stage.

Feel your way in at the edges of sensation if the core of it is too intense, and don't be surprised if a completely different symptom upstages the one you've chosen to focus on. I have found myself attempting to explore the shape of a headache only to find that fatigue and brain fog were the overwhelming voices, clouding out the details of the pain even as its overall structure loomed large.

The voice of my illness is...

Does a name or persona present itself to you when you start the above sentence? What descriptors come to mind? Write as many different endings to the sentence 'The voice of my illness is...' as feel appropriate to you, using any of the words in the box if you need a kickstart.

> Fragile Lupine Authoritative Striped Confused Red Solid
> Scratchy Heavy Loud Mercurial Fluid Afraid Protective
> Cruel Secretive Foreign Hot Clear Hesitant Caring
> Bitter Safe Young Hostile Antiseptic Unique Wise
> Amorphous Spiky Contradictory Gentle Deceptive Wavy
> Alarmed Elusive Dull Defensive Blurred Bright Busy

Suggested therapeutic activity

From debris to declaration

Investigate whether you could be inspired by the detritus of healthcare. Use a familiar item associated with living with your illness to give a voice to your condition or to the parts of you affected by it. You might embroider or paint relevant words on well-used bedding or compression stockings. Maybe copies of medical letters, torn up and rearranged will convey something previously unexpressed. I enjoyed creating a piece that involved re-filling the blister pack of my medication with representations of better times returning – beach sand, a tiny shell, a silver star, dried petals and leaves, musical notes cut from sheet music, a sunflower seed, a heart-shaped button and more. I called it Modern Magic and included the text, 'Side-effects of this medicine may include seeds of hope, many-petalled joys, a held together heart and reconnection with the music of life.'

Listening to the voice of illness at a glance

- Rather than attempting to block out unpleasant sensations, listen attentively to the raw, unfiltered voice of the experience, for a while, as a way into a potential body of work.
- What is the tone, speech pattern or message of your illness or a prominent symptom? You can exorcise, counterbalance, explore or celebrate this in your creative acts.
- Employ alternative sensations to translate and depict difficult-to-portray symptoms.
- If you were a professional sculptor, poet, architect or chef, etc., how would you portray your illness or a key symptom?
- Hypersensitivity and other symptoms can enhance your descriptive powers and lend their voices to artistic visions.
- Discarded paraphernalia of chronic illness make interesting art materials.

Chapter 24
Maximising your environment

Your environment is likely limited by your condition. You may be mostly housebound, even fully bedbound. For some, even their window onto the world is obscured by the curtains and blinds that protect them from the pain of sunlight.

Unable to take your senses far afield, how can you bring some of that gloriously inspiring world to you? When chronically ill our home becomes our retreat, our studio, our uplift and downtime, the backdrop for celebrations and a place of mundane routine. It is our daily canvas or manuscript paper, if you will. We can use this environment and the objects within it to consistently replenish our well of creativity.

I take William Morris's advice to 'Have nothing in your houses that you do not know to be beautiful or believe to be useful' and lead it a step further by aiming to fill my environment only with things that qualify on both these counts simultaneously. If I'm to be captive in this environment, I intend to make it my house of delights.

> *If I'm to be captive in this environment, I intend to make it my house of delights.*

Fill your living space with anything that stimulates your creativity. Natural objects, evocative art, textiles, artists' materials to play with, music and musical instruments, if so inclined. Have mood boards and pinboards and inspiration walls. It has been suggested that the more restricted by her health that Frida Kahlo became the more she sought to bring the natural world into her domain, welcoming plants and animals into her home to enhance her life and her connection with the outside world. We can't all look after living creatures or maintain houseplants, but we can consider how to enrich the space we are forced to spend most of our time in.

'The physician heals, nature makes well,' Aristotle said, and so, along with houseplants and herbs and tumbled gemstones that I can roll in my palm, I have feathers and shells and driftwood, water-pocked pebbles and other *objets trouvés* arranged in my rooms. These are tactile items that can be appreciated through the sense of touch when eyes are shut or light is dimmed. Some were collected on better days that allowed for excursions, holding memories in their bodies, others have been brought to me by friends and family. Keeping such natural treasures company in my home are my textile re-creations of fungi, stitched butterflies and felted leaves. If I can't get out into the wilderness then, whenever able, I will create a version of it to live with me.

Libby is a mixed-media artist whose chronic condition allows her to leave the house to take local photographs of the natural world and collect ingredients for her creativity. Once back home, she makes ink from nuts, rust and other natural substances. The great outdoors is brought into her sanctuary to make a home with her, not just through the images she paints but the materials they are painted with. In a similar way, your environment can welcome other locations into its embrace. Photographs and representations of nature adorn my walls, along with artwork that I have created through the combination of stitch, pressed leaves and flowers, and natural imagery.

An extra illusory dimension can be added with judicious use of windows, mirrors and scenic pictures to bring new stimuli and distant dreams closer. Being fortunate enough to tolerate sunlight, I have banished the veil of net curtains and watch the way light and shadows affect colours, cast patterns and soften or sharpen lines in the room. Mirrors positioned to reflect more of the outside into my sedentary viewpoint also bounce light around while stealing extra views from outside to increase my horizons and blur the boundaries of my confinement. Meanwhile, landscape paintings and photographs, as well as depictions of fantasy worlds and maps, lead you into their depths, sparking imaginative journeys. The author Claire Wade says that she 'started having a music stand by my bed, holding an open book of art, when I was first bedbound. It meant I could look at different pictures every day, like an ever-changing window or gallery of my own.'

Having said all this, I also offer the seemingly contradictory advice to declutter when able. My saxophone, oil paints and some textiles that I had to accept couldn't be used by me have been passed on. Clearing out and swapping around is as much a way of maximising stimulation from the environment we're used to as introducing new items. Treasures may emerge through fresh placement, while clean lines and space will draw your attention towards the carefully selected clusters of interest. Give peaceful attention to engaging in the curation and arrangement of your belongings, just as you would any other creative act.

It may be that minimalism is where you feel most comfortable. If this is the case, ensure that whatever finds itself honoured enough to be in your space truly deserves its position. Be sure it creatively nourishes you. Your selection of inspirations may be held within one cupboard that opens its doors onto a creative wonderland, or a piece of technology that allows you to attend virtual tours, view exhibitions and experience 360-degree photographs from around the world. Through the internet you can peruse online antique, charity and art supply shops for ideas; discover reams of luxury fabrics from which you can absorb patterns and colourways; and introduce yourself to all manner of creative influences without moving more than your fingers or your voice.

The closer you look, the more is revealed.

When feelings of regret that you can't explore more actively inevitably arise, seek to discover more in your own curve of the world with whatever you can welcome into it. The coastline paradox refers to the fact that the length of a coastline will be different depending on the method of measurement and the scale being used. This is due to the fractal nature of coastlines. The closer you study them the more bays and curves and inlets and bends reveal themselves and the longer the coastline becomes, *ad infinitum*. You may not have a view of a coastline from your sickroom, but the same rule applies: the closer you look, the more is revealed. Study the skin of a piece of fruit, the detailing on a curtain, the shadows of the creases in the drape of fabric, the architecture of a crack in the wall, the brushwork in a painting. Can you see echoes of the vastness of the universe in the small environment you occupy? By narrowing your vision down to the microcosm, does more become available to you?

Suggested creative exercises
Micro-vision

Using a piece of card or sturdy paper, cut a 5-10 cm square in the centre. Discard the square and use the cut-out window as a frame to look through. Hold it up, viewing what you can see through this miniature window, or place it on the surface of an object (a brick, floor tile, marrow, scrap of cloth, piece of wood or tree bark, pile of leaves, bunch of ripening bananas, etc.) and depict only what is revealed in this small, framed square. What colours, patterns, textures or miniature worlds can you perceive that had gone unrecognised when gazing at the overall view? Expand what your senses can draw upon by observing in this way the finer details of the mundane.

Altering your environment

Choose a way to experiment with altering your experience of a familiar environment. Pick one of the following suggestions or try any ideas of your own:
- Put your pillows at the foot of the bed and lie or sleep with your feet where your head would normally rest.
- Leave the curtains open when the sun sets and fully experience the change in light and atmosphere.
- If you have a spare bedroom that you don't often occupy, lie in there. Take a holiday away from your bed for a night.

- Play nature sounds – a burbling river, birdsong, crashing waves, a crackling fire. (Meditation apps are great for providing a selection of ambient sounds.)
- Sit in the garden at night.
- Create space where there is clutter.
- Decorate a utilitarian object.
- Rearrange displays or the way you organise possessions.
- Periodically change photographs or pictures in frames.
- Turn electric lights off and light candles instead. (If the flickering of a candle flame is uncomfortable, light more than one so that their individual flickers are balanced out by each other's movement and stillness.)
- Lie on the floor and examine how different perspectives and details come into play.
- View your surroundings through a mirror.
- Light incense or burn essential oils that evoke a different atmosphere
- Watch the smoke rising off a joss stick.

Suggested therapeutic activity

Creating an altar

An altar needn't just be for the religious or spiritually minded. It is simply a dedicated space that feeds your spirit. You could use the top of a chest of drawers, a coffee table in the corner of the room, or a shelf on the wall. You might even think of a noticeboard as your version of an altar. If you're really pushed for space, create a virtual altar via your digital device, a world-building computer game or good old-fashioned drawing.

Dedicate this space to something that will enhance the time you spend in this environment and bring something new to you, simultaneously exploring and honouring your creativity. You could use it to welcome into your environment places that you are unable to visit, filling it with representations of a particular destination or having a nature altar that brings the outside world indoors to you. You may choose to focus on a colour palette inspired by a photograph, or the many hues and tones of one colour. Perhaps your altar will be dedicated to a particular artist. Or maybe you will adorn it traditionally with images of deities or saints – Brigid, Celtic goddess and Christian saint of poetry, healing and smithcraft; Saraswati, Hindu goddess of the arts, nature and music; Minerva, Roman goddess of healing, music, inspiration and handicrafts, especially weaving; Athena, Greek goddess of the arts, especially weaving; Hephaestus, Greek jewellery-crafting god who taught the importance of making art in all its forms and used the taunts he received about his limp as a catalyst for his art; Saint Luke, patron saint of doctors and artists.

Change the focus or some of the contents of your altar as often as you feel the need to welcome fresh input into the space you inhabit.

Maximising your environment at a glance

- Make your environment a microcosm of the wider world you want to inhabit.
- Bring the outdoors in through pictures, mirrors, plants, found treasures and crafted re-creations.
- Consider how practical items that you require around you can be more aesthetically pleasing or creatively enhanced.
- Arranging objects for display can have a similarly calming effect on the brain as other creative acts.
- When space is at a premium, use folders (on a device or actual stationery folders) to store a multitude of images.
- Use the internet to widen your world.
- Change what you surround yourself with. Pictures, soft furnishings and dedicated altars can be adjusted with the seasons or other time spans.
- Look more closely at what is around you and discover greater detail.

Chapter 25
Flights of fancy

Florence Nightingale reported seeing patients denied living plants or glasses of cut flowers by nurses who considered these bedside items unhealthy. She also observed how the cravings of the sick for colour and variety were dismissed by nurses as their 'fancies'. Far from being fanciful, she believed these longings were an indication of what could aid recovery. Fanciful desires are often sanity savers, allowing us moments of escapist respite, along the plodding and precipitous path of chronic illness.

A fanciful imagination is an enriching quality that many delving into creativity would love to possess more of. Chronic illness, in many ways, offers a fertile environment to develop this trait. To an extent, we are removed from daily normality and the automatic responses to a busy life. We see the world a little askance – from a wheelchair rather than standing height, from a generally prone position, from the perspective of someone who must regularly adapt to ever-changing needs or whose senses over-react to stimuli. Forced to rest for lengths of time, our eyes seek creatures in the shadows on the wall and faces in the knots of furniture wood.

Anything can be worthy of inspiration. How can you interpret what's around you imaginatively? Use all your senses, a variety of perspectives, and think metaphorically. Follow wherever your imagination leads, regardless of how foolish, inane or bizarre it may seem. Flights of fancy are where originality is born.

Xavier De Maistre, not confined due to ill health but under house arrest in the eighteenth century, did just this when he wrote his parody of a travelogue, *A*

Voyage Around My Room. 'What a comfort the new mode of travelling will be to the sick,' he wrote. 'In this room which we travel ... no obstacle shall hinder our way and giving ourselves up gaily to Imagination, we will follow her whithersoever it may be her good pleasure to lead us.' Like De Maistre, let your mind make new terrain of your familiar surroundings. I have been known to liken my stair-lift to a ski-lift or a (disappointingly slow) fairground ride.

Take an imaginative approach to routines you have engaged in countless times. A much looked-forward-to shower becomes a tropical waterfall pouring over us, the steam in the bathroom recreating the humid atmosphere of distant climes, or the scent of clean water taking us back to a holiday pool. In this way our spirit is rejuvenated, and our mind is led to thoughts and memories that can stimulate fresh creativity.

Craft a creative mind-set and fly further in your mind.

If your own belongings or surroundings aren't offering up inspiration, trawl the internet for unusual items, stimulating images and evocative sounds that awaken new, fantastical thought-paths. Absorb fantasy, folklore and science fiction, if these appeal. Look on estate agents' or holiday accommodation websites and imagine who, or what, might live in these abodes. Whether or not you produce anything tangible with these ideas is irrelevant. You are crafting a creative mind-set and learning to fly further in your mind.

Our bodies may feel trapped in illness but perhaps our minds can soar free for a while, bringing back souvenirs to work with. Imagining is a creative and life-affirming act that our amygdala (that primal, reactive part of our brain) has trouble discerning from reality. Imagine something enough and part of our being accepts that it has really happened, so let's take a running jump off the cliff of reality and glide on unadulterated fantasy.

Being predominantly bedbound with severe ME, endometriosis and post-operative colitis can be extra hard for Katie when the sun is shining, or her partner has gone on a well-deserved holiday. To help herself in these situations

Chapter 25

she has collected a folder of destinations she knows she'll never visit in real life but can travel to in her mind. Her health limits how she can express her creative side but just gathering these idyllic images and arranging them in a folder is a creative act that feeds her inner self. When brain fog inhibits her power to conjure fantasy destinations, she is prepared with an armoury of imagery.

> *Imagining is a creative and life-affirming act.*

'I have an imaginary island with different visualisation spaces inspired by pictures I've found,' Katie explains. 'There's a cove, a breezy clifftop, a bluebell wood, a stream, a jungle treehouse, a log cabin with a real fire, a wildflower meadow, a field of tulips and lots of twisty paths leading to new, unexplored places.' She doesn't concern herself with practicalities of environmental proximities or access, but simply travels with the whims of desire. She also plays videos found on YouTube of exotic scenes, regarding the screen as a window onto a holiday location. During a heatwave, without absconding from bed, a beach with waves crashing onto a white-sanded shore – the breeze ruffling palm leaves under a cerulean sky and drifting clouds – carries her afar. Uniting the weather and technology in this way not only sets a respite scene for you to fall into, but potentially evokes more detailed creative inspiration while you're there.

Inspired by Holidays from Home, a concept created by Claire Wade when her health prevented her from joining her family on their summer holiday, fanciful flights that I've indulged in have included a day trip to Tuscany (plenty of Italian food was consumed and the fields of sunflowers were evoked with supermarket-delivered sunflowers); scuba diving in Belize (shells, sea salt, a snorkel and swimwear, all in the bath); and a Home Sweet Home festival (complete with author interviews and readings via YouTube, silent disco for my husband, food marquee and pamper pod). Our honeymoon was a virtual world tour that took place over a week without either of us leaving the house. Each day we experienced a different country through food, drink, music, viewing material and items of traditional clothing. Contrary to my fears that my husband was being deprived of a 'real' honeymoon, he still talks, over a decade on, about the atmosphere created, the fun we had and the 'postcards' we shared via social media.

Organising such events is a creative act that mustn't be underrated. We printed out an itinerary complete with photographs of 'destinations', music playlists, location-appropriate films and menus. Flight boarding cards were made, local card games and board games suggested, real hotels found online that we wanted to imagine staying at, and props were acquired to immerse us in the event.

I have also attended an online ball organised by a housebound member of the chronic illness community who wanted to celebrate a special birthday and was willing to employ creative writing, borrowed images (oh, the ballgowns we chose from!) and imaginative thought to enjoy herself. How can you integrate the flights you fancy into your creative life? Where would you like to go, what fantasies would you like to dally with, and how can you honour that desire where you are? To misquote Lisa St Aubin De Teran from a short story of hers: truant from your sick bed.

One of the most successful times for absenting from illness and embarking on flights of fancy is sleep and that liminal hinterland on the outskirts of it (insomnia and symptom-soaked dreams, aside). Whether it is my condition, the medication I require or a combination of the two that ramps up the technicolour memorability of my dreams I don't know, but any lack of physical adventures or imaginative inspiration in my waking hours is rarely experienced when I sleep. In something akin to vivid hallucinations and fever dreams, stunning horizons, surreal juxtapositions, beautiful fragrances and clearly heard melodies greet me. The nightmares are just as powerful, causing me to wake shouting, hitting out and sodden with sweat, but even these are valuable sources of darker inspiration. My nocturnal flights seemingly know no bounds and for this I'm thankful. Even when I know my dreamscapes to be figments of fancy, the sensations and concepts reside with me, wanting to outlive their natural habitat.

We are so used to living with ourselves that we don't always recognise our strengths and gifts. I spent years both marvelling at the intricate lucidity of my dreams and simultaneously bemoaning a lack of ideas and plot lines for story writing. It finally dawned on me that my mind had been providing what I sought all along. When I decided to embrace the snapshots and inconclusive nature of my night-world, I found they had much to offer my writing. One dream from my early teens impressed itself on me as being story worthy but I couldn't fathom a clear destination for the plot. The dream had ended abruptly, never to be revisited and I couldn't discover a resolution. Some 30 years later, I realised that the lack of a conclusion could be incorporated as a poignant aspect of the story. I made my younger self very happy the day I finally turned that dream into a piece of flash fiction.

The Tboli women of southern Mindanao in the Philippines believe that the patterns they weave into the textile they call *t'nalak* are delivered to them in their dreams by the goddess Fu Dalo. It is to this guardian spirit that they turn for inspiration, rather than any prescribed or handed down designs, and thus they are known as 'dreamweavers'. What mementos can you bring back from your night- and daydreams to enrich your creative endeavours?

> *We are so used to living with ourselves that we don't always recognise our strengths. It finally dawned on me that my mind had been providing what I sought all along.*

Suggested creative exercises

Dream journal

Keep a journal of anything you want to remember from your dreams, employing whatever format most appeals to you. Your journal might be as disjointed and chaotic as your dreamworld, inhabited by random words, phrases in speech bubbles, line drawings, surreal images and descriptive paragraphs. There may be narrative or pure imagery, splashes of colour or dark scribbles that evoke wordless feelings. You might choose to create a stitched dream journal, embroidering a choice image or word each day from the previous night (or day-nap). Or perhaps it will be an audio journal. Have fun using this space to preserve the concoctions of your subconscious, either as expressive art or as a repository for potential inspiration.

Finding a fanciful companion (or exorcising a demon)

For this exercise you will need a piece of paper large enough for you to make relaxed movements on it with a pencil. With your eyes closed and pencil in hand (your non-dominant hand if you want to make even less predictable shapes), doodle without lifting the pencil from the paper. Move your hand around without thought or inhibition. When you feel ready, open your eyes and look for what can be found in the shapes you've created. Go over lines that lend themselves to being outlines of a creature. Add extra details, erase lines that have become superfluous and let the patterns on the page feed your imagination until you've created a fanciful being, a mythical hybrid, a guardian spirit or the soul of your sickness. Allow it to emerge however your fancy suggests. No concerted effort or precise motor skills are needed to reveal all manner of images hiding within random lines and shapes.

You may want to leave it as a simple line-drawing or develop the idea further. Colour it in with precision or use watercolour paints loosely over the image without staying within the lines for a more ethereal feel. Create a story involving this character or make a textile toy or puppet. Ask it how it would like to grow, and go on a flight of fancy with it,

Suggested therapeutic activity
Postcards from another reality

Take yourself on a journey in your mind, or played out at home; then, through photography, drawing, painting, sewing, text, stock images, digital art, etc., create a postcard from this fantasy destination. Indulge your dreams and bring them at least partially into being. This postcard can be for yourself or sent to another who will understand the need for a missive from another reality. Some ideas for destinations to send your postcards from include:
- The past
- The future
- Inside a favourite book, film, painting or poem

- A luxury spa day (courtesy of a mobile massage service, your bath, a soft robe and a face mask, if you want to enact this flight of fancy)
- A virtual holiday (literally anywhere in the world)
- Outer space
- Deep inner space
- A dream
- An alternative universe in which you and the people you know inhabit different roles and abilities.

Flights of fancy at a glance

- A little of what you fancy does you good – even when so much of what you fancy is denied you. What fancies can you explore through imaginative thought and creative expression?
- A fanciful imagination is a healthy coping mechanism when feeling trapped.
- Use the circumstances that long-term illness presents you with to let your mind wander further into unusual perspectives.
- Don't be afraid to be odd, silly or different. These are creative attributes.
- Everyday objects can inspire fanciful responses. One room can become a metaphor for a global journey. One item can inspire a creative response.
- Imaginary events, travels and experiences are felt by your amygdala as if they have really happened. Planning and enjoying virtual excursions for yourself and others is a creatively fulfilling act.
- Dreams are a doorway into fantastical worlds. Keeping a dream diary may help you remember more of them to bring back with you as creative fodder.
- In flights of fancy, you can be whoever and wherever you like. Express your essence through your imagination.

Chapter 26
Borrowing from others

Lucy Perillo, the nature-loving poet who lived the end of her life with degenerative multiple sclerosis (MS), observed how easy it is to become so focused on our personal drama that we can become detached from the world beyond ourselves. She wrote about the self being a poem that is limited by this exclusion of wider experiences. How can we help the world to enter our cloistered realm when our health guards the entry points so closely? We look to borrow from others and smuggle in what we can. Smuggling may involve reading small snippets of whole texts, listening just to the music that can be heard by you and not your body's alarm system, or engaging with other artists and crafters in ways that sneak under your condition's radar. In whatever capacity your body can tolerate, I encourage you to revel in other people's creativity, in their lived experiences and their explorations.

Borrow widely from diverse influences. Absorb as much as you can from different cultures and voices. Listen to perspectives that diverge from your own. Travel into other minds through podcasts, audiobooks, blogs, online articles, magazines, children's books, novels, memoirs and non-fiction. Open books at random (library books, cheap second-hand books, favourite inhabitants of your own bookshelves…) and dip in and out of them like delicious tapas for the mind.

Dip in and out of diverse influences like delicious tapas for the mind.

You are not looking to plagiarise but to absorb creativity by osmosis. Remind yourself how you feel around creativity and let it all percolate. Flit between perspectives and approaches, honing what you want to express and how you could achieve this. Watch films, documentaries and craft programmes. Listen to a variety of music genres, learn about traditions from around the world, peruse online galleries and museum tours. Tuck away snippets of other people's poetry and sparkling glimpses of life and see how they rearrange themselves in your sleep.

Borrow, scavenge and tweak from an array of artists, disciplines, traditions and areas of life. Follow creative people or those who deliver new experiences to you on social media. Research any creators who pique your interest. Investigate their influences, muses and role models. Gather your inspiration and techniques indiscriminately, cross-referencing skills until you find what works well for you. Borrow a theme, subject matter or plot and transpose it into an entirely different medium, turning a painting into a poem, perhaps, or a character from mythology into a cartoon caricature or handcrafted doll.

Austin Kleon, author of *Steal Like An Artist*, asserts that it's not another's style you're seeking to take for yourself but the way of thinking or behaving that led to that style. Establish the tonal qualities that you want to honour and work out how they have been achieved, developing a connection with the process before progressing to uncovering your own original version. Ask yourself why you like the things that appeal to you and what it is about other creations that jar with you. Is there a common factor? Find patterns in your likes and dislikes to discover where you want to focus your creative energy. Ask yourself why you feel the way you do about something. Go deeper. Here will lie the essence of your creative urge, resting beneath any kneejerk desire to duplicate another's artistry.

If able, take part in online courses, classes, creativity challenges or craft-alongs. Join crafty online groups where ideas can be bounced around, picking up and shedding suggestions as they find their rightful creator. Ask others for creativity prompts, titles or launch-words to bypass your habitual thought patterns. The more creativity we are exposed to, the more likely we are to feel inspirationally invigorated.

Steal patterns and rhythms and colour combinations from nature. Look to other species, even plants and minerals, for behaviours or viewpoints to borrow. If you can't get out, piggyback on other people's adventures. Encourage healthy people to 'take you with them' via photographs or videos of their excursions and holidays.

The more creativity we are exposed to, the more likely we are to feel inspirationally invigorated.

To some this may feel like rubbing salt in the wound of your confinement, but I find that when the person has captured the scenery with me in mind I feel as if a part of me has been there with them. 'I photographed this plant because it struck me as one you'd like,' said one friend while bringing to my living room as much as she could of the rainforest biome of Cornwall's Eden Project. The simple act of having been included by thought takes the sting out of not being able to travel in person and enables me to benefit from the experience vicariously.

Fill your mind with as great a variety of input to sift through and choose from as possible. Once you have borrowed what appeals to you from other people's exposure and responses to the world, you can then tilt it all to your own slant. At what angle do you experience the world that has been brought to you? How does it touch you, having passed through the filters of longing, dizziness, dimmed light, tinnitus, anxiety, pain, hope, recollection, appreciation, wonder, acceptance, imagination?

Suggested creative exercises

Borrow some style

Replicate as closely as you can a piece of art or craftwork that you admire. Don't claim it as your own original design – this is an exercise not in plagiarism but in learning how to reproduce qualities that will enhance your own work. Absorb how the process feels to your hands and other senses. Trace a line drawing; follow a textile pattern to the letter; copy a section of a painting or the style of marks made by a revered artist; handwrite a beloved poem or type a chapter written by a favourite author. Get a practical feel for the characteristics you want to include in your work before trying out your own interpretation of the style.

Take something, anything

Create a collage from portions of other people's work. By the time you've finished, the components you use will be like the ingredients in a recipe – none dominating the flavour but all working together to create the sensory feast. Your collage may be formed from cut or torn sections of printed out artworks, from craft magazine pictures, from words lifted from a vast array of texts. It may be a patchwork of embroidered scraps, a musical montage, a story or poem created from a multitude of first (or last) lines of novels. Perhaps you will choose an existing piece of artwork, literature, craft kit or pattern and take it apart, move the pieces around and make a mosaic of the original elements. Credit the original sources and give the final piece a name that reflects your treatment of them.

Suggested therapeutic activity

Borrowing from the old and often told

In her online master class, Margaret Atwood proposes leading a classic folktale in a new direction by writing a fresh opening for it. If I were to choose Little Red Riding Hood, for example, I might open with the line: 'She knew the villagers referred to Grandma's sickness as The Wolf'.

Use your chosen discipline to recreate or adapt a borrowed plotline, theme, character, event, poem, scene or quote. Borrow from myth, legend, folklore, classic literature, your own history or anyone else's (due discretion considered!). Carol Ann Duffy's poetry collection *The World's Wife*, for example, consists of poems told in the imagined voices of female counterparts to well-known fictional and factual male characters. Borrow from any source that ignites a desire to represent it in a new light, different genre, fresh style or alternative perspective; perhaps with an original twist or personal take on the subject matter.

Take what has been shared, repeated, bowdlerised or embellished and reclaim it for this present moment; for yourself.

Borrowing from others at a glance

- Welcome fresh perspectives and a wide array of influences into your awareness.
- Borrow from flora and fauna, not just other people.
- Television documentaries, radio programmes, podcasts, art books, postcards, poetry, audiobooks, fiction, world religion, history, memoir, online museums and galleries – these all broaden our minds and therefore our creative output.
- Store up heard experiences.
- Pay attention to techniques that other creatives use in their work.
- When something moves you, ask yourself what it is that is specifically affecting you so that you can incorporate this effect into your own work.
- Encourage others to 'take you with them' when they visit interesting places, by taking photographs, short videos, or voiced narratives specifically to share with you.
- Borrow themes, structures or isolated aspects of well-known art or historical events to instigate your own creative exploration.

Chapter 27
Contradictions and combinations

Whether we know it or not, we seek contrast and balance for a satisfying, exciting or thought-provoking experience. Creative projects, therefore, require either instinctive or considered combinations and contradictions for the most effective results. 'I'm only knitting a scarf,' you may say. But the colours, textures and stitches you choose all contribute to the visual and textural interest and appeal. There is always room to investigate how we can best combine and contrast in our creations.

Whether you are a fan of freedom and movement in your work, enjoying creative licence and a loose effect, or are more at home with methodical structure and tradition, challenge yourself to look to the opposite of your status quo. Don't ignore your personal style but do consider how the reverse of your regular practice could benefit your aims or rejuvenate your creative mojo. Would a combined approach enable you to take your work further, either physically or artistically?

The designer Donatella Versace believes that creativity surfaces from a conflict of ideas. Anyone with a desire to do something but not the means to do it will know that conflicting needs are just as influential. 'A need or problem encourages creative efforts,' declared Plato. When negotiating chronic illness, attention to the fine balance between conflicting pulls on our resources is crucial. We must maintain a healthy pathway between concentration and relaxation, activity and rest, advance and consolidation. A life that smoothly combines the contrasting needs of an active creator with a chronically ill person is a finely woven creation in itself. And, like all weavings, we wouldn't be what we are without the interconnected directions of the opposing warp and weft threads.

Tension and resolution combine in a repeating pattern that stimulates enthusiasm and the endorphin rush of success. Enthusiasm itself is paired with the more plodding partner of dispirited uncertainty and together they move under, over, up and down, forwards, backwards and forwards again. Sometimes outright contradiction is exactly what we need to address.

So, to achieve more, what might you include less of? Do you ironically make greater progress when you work for shorter periods of time, discovering creative solutions and leaps of insight after you've stepped away from the work? Do your paintings look more interesting when you pare back the brush strokes or omit certain details? Do you elicit stronger understanding around your illness when you forego depictions of the multitudinous symptoms or concerns to instead focus on just one, giving the responder the opportunity to connect more intimately? Conversely, what might you include more of to draw attention to its opposite? Does the light in your drawings shine clearer when you add more shade and darkness around it? Do delicate hues sing brighter against colours that you might have feared too dark to include? Do you better communicate the limitations of your body when you highlight the things it does rather than list what you can't do? Always be on the lookout for how strategically putting more weight elsewhere may draw greater attention to where you want the focus to be.

Disorder within a clearly delineated space feels uninhibited without communicating poor skill.

Similarly, in the physical act of creating, can that which you've been trying to overcome instead be harnessed and drawn attention to? Instead of inhibiting you, does following your body's lead when it contradicts your intentions hold the potential to enhance the outcome? If you struggle to focus your eyes or use tools with precision, how can the results of these difficulties be included rather than bemoaned or binned?

Experiment with combining careful composition with aspects of chaos and surprise so that, by using form and structure to contain or offset irregularity, you can deliver a sense of liberation or anarchy in a way that is received coherently. Disorder within a clearly delineated space, for example, feels uninhibited without communicating confusion or poor skill.

Play with all kinds of combinations and contradictions and how they interact with each other. Too many all at once will bicker and shout, creating a muddle, but look for the ones that spark an interesting conversation with each other and follow these. Try combining images or ideas from the natural world with manmade objects. Integrate the wild and the tamed, the modern and the traditional, the healthy and problematic aspects of yourself. Merge organic forms with angular shapes. Mix genres and materials. Crochet with wire, draw with makeup, embroider on paper or dried leaves. Sit the mundane with the magical, the flouncy with the stark, the scientific with the ethereal, the past with the future, monochrome with technicolour. Make the practical delightful. Give the sublime a job.

None of this is an instruction to make Frankenstein art – unless that is your intent. You don't want to include pretentious contrasts merely for the sake of being different, but do remain open to fresh combinations. Be willing to dissolve any soluble boundaries presented by your health, regular materials or habitual thought patterns.

When solving an anagram, I move the letters into all kinds of random combinations before finding the hidden word. I know that where I'm placing the letters isn't yet going to yield the answer but that the fresh juxtapositions will lead me to it. Employing the same technique with more creative endeavours – moving items around, aligning apparently unrelated concepts, objects and words with each other, collating disparate patterns, colours and methods – will often point me in an interesting direction. It doesn't matter how many times you 'fail' to create something pleasing. All these movements are potential steps on the way to a creative epiphany. Playing around may feel like procrastination or frippery but, despite its indirect nature, it is often one of the most direct routes to inspiration's abode. Play and work needn't be the contradiction that these words imply. Epiphany or not, playing without aim is part of creative work.

Similarly, like and dislike needn't entirely contradict each other. The two can synthesize to produce a work of depth and interest. I have heard it said that every piece of art should provide the observant mind with the space to move between like and dislike. The same is true of living with long-term health conditions. It's a given that you don't like the pain and struggles but what about the rare gifts your condition offers as compensation?

Examine the relationship between like and dislike in your work and see where this takes you.

Looking with interest at the complexity of your situation can stimulate new ways to express yourself in your art. What are the contrasts between the illness as its own entity and you the carrier of it? Does it cause your life to contradict your desires? What does the combination of your condition and your own nature create? Has being chronically ill instigated anything that you might not otherwise have encountered or brought into being? How does putting what you dislike into your creations affect your style? Were you to not worry about whether others like or dislike your work, would you do anything differently? Our work will likely provoke contrasting reactions in others, anyway. It's not something we can control. So, feel free to examine and play with the relationship between like and dislike in your work and see where this takes you.

Clinging to expectations, habits or disappointments crushes creativity. If an idea isn't coming to fruition, ask yourself if something else entirely is trying to emerge, either in its own right or combined with elements of your original plan. When stuck in a creative block or limitation of your body, consider whether you are posing the right questions. Is what you are asking of yourself necessary? Are you looking in the most helpful direction or could a contradictory perspective reveal an entirely new solution? What new angle could you approach the problem from to reveal your solution? What can you combine that hadn't previously occurred to you? When something seems cluttered, does adding more improve it? When something looks unfinished does removing an element bring it to a conclusion? How can you move into a contrasting direction of creative flow?

Explore the possibilities held in the contradictions of your assumptions. Instead of a reflexive 'I can't', spend time with a considered 'How can'? 'I can't paint' becomes: 'How can I creatively express myself?' or: 'How I can recreate the pleasure I used to get from painting?'

Be curious. What if this were big instead of small; rough instead of smooth; patterned instead of plain; short instead of long? What if an inanimate object became animated? Practise the art of questioning the status quo to reveal the artistic, imaginative, and adaptive adventures hiding in unusual syntheses and contradictory pathways.

 **Suggested creative exercises**

Random connections

Use an online random word generator to conjure two unrelated words. Alternatively, open any book with your eyes shut, placing your finger anywhere on the exposed pages. Open your eyes to reveal an arbitrary word and repeat for the second word. Use your randomly selected words to inspire a single piece of writing or artwork. If all you produce is one paragraph or a loosely sketched surreal line-drawing, that's fine. Use this exercise to loosen up your mind and encourage it to make original connections. Here are some random word pairings to get you started:

Decision/Tin	Noon/Pearl	Reflection/Apricot
Fairies/Comparison	Smell/Spy	Victory/Grudge
Moon/Tongue	Nail/Smile	Seashore/Cloth
Desire/Branch	Dirt/Recognition	Spice/Watch

Yin and yang

List any three things you like or admire and three that you dislike or find no merit in. These can be objects, hobbies, people, books, food – anything – but try to include at least one piece of art or craftwork in each list. Take time to consider the specifics that you appreciate in your liked items and what it is that repels you in your disliked items.

Now, investigate whether you have any ambivalent feelings about these items. Are there aspects of your liked items that you're not keen on, or components of your disliked items that you find interesting or pleasant or that are objectively successful? How do these co-exist and possibly augment each other? What pitfalls have you identified that you will avoid in your own work and what successful traits have you isolated that you might learn from? Like the image of the yin-yang, do these contradictions contain the seeds of each other inside themselves? Discover more about your personal tastes, and the relationship between positive and negative associations and responses.

Suggested therapeutic activity
Combining contradictory views

You may like to use this activity for the benefit of your artwork or as an opportunity to reframe something about your health condition that you usually struggle with. This is not to negate how you feel, but an exercise in recognising new possibilities.

Choose an object, sensation, emotion or symptom to write three pieces about. Depending on your energy levels and inclination, these can be anything from a selection of words, phrases or a single sentence to poems or essays.

In your first piece aim to be objectively descriptive, remaining neutral in your descriptors. Avoid any imagery that suggests a positive or negative slant.

Chapter 27

For the second piece, depict your chosen subject with the reverse filter of your instinctive perception. Remain true to your senses' experiences but reframe where your focus lies to deliver an entirely different response or atmosphere. Contradict your habitual response, setting your subject in a new light for this exercise. This may require you imagining you are someone or something else entirely and how that entity would perceive your subject matter.

And now, for the third piece, use some or all of what you have already written as a launch pad for a piece of writing (or alternative creation) that combines neutral observations with your natural perceptions as well as more considered explorations into the contradictory reactions you have elicited. Experiment with novel imagery, including associations and emotive descriptors that may seem at odds with each other, to produce a more holistic depiction.

Practising this widening of perception may help you to convey something you usually struggle to say about living with ill health or to respond to the world around you, in any creative genre, with greater originality.

Contradictions and combinations at a glance

- Contrast and balance are important components of creative work.
- Play with mixing things up, combining different styles, and contradicting the expected.
- A conflict of ideas results in greater creativity when explored and merged.
- Pay attention to conflicts of need in your own life and how you can balance these within your creative hobbies.
- Less can be more. To make something more complete, perhaps something could be removed.
- Alternatively, something you thought finished but are dissatisfied with may need adding to. In this case, building the piece up may be the answer.
- Light requires darkness to be recognised for its brightness. Remember to include depth of shade in your work (metaphorically or literally).
- Emphasising something's opposite can draw people's attention to where you really want the focus to be.
- Combine different crafts, techniques and concepts.
- Consider allowing both pleasing and jarring elements to bounce off each other in your work, encouraging the viewer to move between these polarities.
- Experiment with contradictory assumptions and see where this takes you.

Chapter 28
Gathering the yarns of your life

Gathering and sharing stories is more natural to us than we may realise. Anecdotes, exaggerations, gossip, fibs, jokes and desires are all yarns we tell. Our physicality, especially, has a narrative to share. In *The Wounded Storyteller*, medical sociologist Arthur Frank points out that an imperative to develop fresh story-paths is initiated by the body itself, when illness unseats the stories you previously lived by.

By attempting to live in a story that has ended, or is paused until the next instalment, you could be depriving yourself of the magic to be found in the current yarn spooling out around you. Life is textured and intricate. Use it with interest even when it feels like the fabric of existence is inhibiting you. Your most difficult times may be the weaving of the raw material that you will come to use creatively.

Be imaginative about what you choose to utilise, transmute or embrace. Gather the different treasures, loose ends and materials found within your body, your mind, your habits, haunts and home. Spin recollections and objects into the yarn that tells of your existence. It may have tangled, meandering, balled up lengths. You might not be able to find the beginning or the end of your yarn, splicing sections from the centre only to discover there are multiple threads wound together that separate when examined or are waiting to be joined together. Whatever you have picked up along the way, or held onto from the start, this is your story for you to unwind, and shape with interest, offering it out to whoever you wish to share it with.

Perhaps the first question to ponder should be: 'What story are you already telling?' Simply by being, you are a protagonist with at least some degree of agency and if you can express yourself in one form or another, then you also get to set the tone of the narrative. While the general plotline of your life might feel out of your hands, you get to portray it in the genre of your choice. Whether you perceive the gathered scenes to be tragic, comic or tragicomic, a battle saga, mystery, tale of self-awareness or a collection of recipes and instructions is up to you. You aren't confined to one category. Choose any that you thrive in; any that nurture a creative response. Magical realism, surrealism, short time-hopping vignettes; portrayal in a minor key, illustrations without words, useful handmade objects representing the tale of who you are – the choice is yours.

> *While the general plotline of your life might feel out of your hands, you get to portray it in the genre of your choice.*

When choosing what tale to tell, remain mindful that stories can harm or heal, bear witness or cast judgement. How do the stories you tell about your life affect you and how can you work with them in your creations to make medicine out of potential poison? Take the story you are already telling and work with it until it more closely resembles the one you want to inhabit. Note that this isn't the same as transforming your life into the adventure or romance you wish of it. It's not about miraculous healing. It is a recognition that you can constructively use what your life has already presented you with. Your job is to listen to the tales calling out from the rabble, decide which you want to give your primary attention to, and lend them the best voice they can use.

As a species, we interpret the world and our experiences of it through storytelling, on a societal and individual level. The stories we most often repeat, to ourselves and others, are the ones we either feel most comfortable with or are still processing. What story do you find yourself returning to over and again, either in your general life or in your creative output? Rather than being concerned that you are repeating yourself or are stuck in a creative rut, consider this your motif or theme and riff on it. While you are revisiting this

Chapter 28

narrative, continue assimilating, exorcising or refining it. 'I took to telling the story of my sufferings, and if the phrases were very beautiful I was so much consoled; I even sometimes forgot my sadness by uttering it,' says Philoctetes in the play of the same name by André Gide.

If, however, you are holding yourself in a painful recollection or outlook, question how you can break free while still inside that story. Turn it inside out. Look out of a different window of it, listen for a previously unregistered perspective. I found it helpful, at one point, to write a story using the anthropomorphised voice of my illness as narrator. Temporarily removing myself from centre stage in my own drama helped me to gain objectivity and discover an original way to share my experience. By extracting a story, examining it with curiosity and choosing how to portray it, you get to gain greater understanding and claim a degree of control over it. It takes up less space proportionately in the outer world than it does inside the confines of your body.

In the pursuit of stories to immerse ourselves in, we must waste nothing. When the present is experiencing an inspirational famine, gather from the past. Our memories are a many-volumed collection of stories we can draw upon. Debussy recognised how he reworked memories into his creativity: 'The sound of the sea, the curve of a horizon, wind in leaves, the cry of a bird leave a manifold impression in us. And suddenly, without our wishing it at all, one of these memories spills from us and finds expression in musical language.'

Use memories, photographs, old work uniforms or activity clothes and revisit these aspects of yourself. Your story has many chapters. Which ones do you want to spend time with? Can you find a thread that runs through them all? Look for opportunities to creatively assert aspects of yourself that have been buried by long-term illness and disability. A career in one of the caring professions may have been lost to you, but perhaps you can make much-needed items to donate to hospitals, schools or refuges. Sift through any disorder and debris to find clues to the stories all around you and form new manifestations of the many chronicles you've inhabited.

If illness has dominated most of your life, then thread your needle with longings and desires. Don't be afraid to claim these for yourself. Honour the different possibilities of your selfhood and engage with them creatively to compensate for being unable to do so literally. Connect childhood ambitions with the present you, forming something to be cherished from the disused and edited text of your life. If fiction is the material most readily available to you, then forget about facts and create a fantasy.

Gathering the yarns of your life isn't just about extracting a memoir or an art series about yourself. Whatever medium you are working in, you are telling a story. If the sum of your creations is a collection of crocheted egg cosies, half-completed craft kits, or vaguely pencilled ideas, these are introductions to, and chapters of, the story that is your life. What stories do you want to honour? The journey of pigment to picture? Of natural fleece to knitted jumper? A story of collective injustice or more personal events and reactions? The histories held in the scraps of fabric that you can make into an heirloom quilt? Anything that has undergone change, or has a past, contains its own story; often more than just one. It is your craft to tease out these yarns and depict them in the presentation of your choice.

Whatever medium you are working in, you are telling a story.

Look around for all the tales, imaginings and histories that have gathered in your presence. Hunt out the bones of stories waiting patiently for you to flesh them out. Sort and sift buttons, beads and sea glass. Untangle and rewind ribbons, yarn and threads. Write up overheard snippets of conversation, stranded words of interest and insistent sentences. As your fingers busy themselves let your mind awaken the sleeping stories. If your chosen materials are rehomed or reclaimed from past purposes, then so much the better. Just imagine the tales they could tell!

Listen to the stories within and all around. How can you release them or reconfigure them, introduce them to new company or cradle them with care? A story needn't always consist of well-crafted words. Sometimes just the act of mentally drafting a personal narrative or imagining a scenario is creative endeavour enough. Sometimes the story will want an illustration or a more figurative approach, with the narrative arc being implicit rather than explicit.

Gather your materials (physical and ephemeral, new and old) like a magpie. When corvids are fed regularly by an individual, they will bring gifts (pebbles, lost marbles, shiny bottle tops) to their benefactor. Your creativity is the same. Nourish it regularly with curiosity and it will deliver treasures to you. It is up to you to recognise them as such and arrange these gifts appreciatively.

Suggested creative exercises
Exploring the hidden narrative

Look around for unexpressed stories you can coax out of the objects you share your home with. Who contributed to their manufacture, and what might their history be? Where was it made and does this evoke any narrative for you? From what materials is it constructed? With this in mind, what might its life have been in a previous incarnation? Who and what has this object previously encountered? The same can be done with plants and flowers around you. Are they native? From where do they originate? How were they used in the past – medically, superstitiously, ceremonially, nutritionally or constructively? What characteristics do they seem to exhibit? Just mulling these questions over in your mind will exercise your creativity and prime you to recognise hidden stories, messages and themes everywhere, supplying a source of entertainment as well as potential inspiration.

A guided visualisation for retrieving stories

Either ask somebody to read this visualisation out for you or record it in advance to play back to yourself.

Make yourself as comfortable as you can and imagine floating in warm water. Feel the ebb and flow of gentle waves supporting you. Just like the waves, inspiration comes and goes but your buoyant creative core is ever-present, keeping you afloat. Stay with this awareness for a while.

Now, step out of the water into a soft robe and warm yourself beside a cosy fire. Notice how the flames leap into animated images and spark ideas in you. Can you feel a link between the embers and the creative fire in your belly? Sometimes it smoulders, at other times it roars. Always, the fire of creativity is within you. Warm yourself with this knowledge.

Now ask the fire what story wants to come forth to be portrayed. Look to the mesmeric movement of the flames for any images your subconscious offers. Take as long as you need for your mind to settle. Let the flames speak for themselves.

In time, you notice a phoenix rising from the dancing images in your mind's eye. Up it flies from the flames, clutching an egg in its claws which it drops on the earth at your feet. As the egg lands it may crack open to reveal the foundation of a story. Anything can emerge from this egg or perhaps nothing at all. Examine what is given to you, even if it is emptiness. Look at it from all angles. Interact with it. How can you nurture it into a fully-fledged story? If it makes no sense to you, or your egg didn't crack open, bury it in the embers of your creative fire to gestate a little longer.

Tell the contents of the egg that you are committed to finding out how to share its story. Can you see whether its structure will be audible, tactile or visual? Is it fictional, factual or a blend of the two? Visualise how you will feel when you have brought it into being. Absorb the sensation of achieving your aim.

Now take a moment to consider how you have already begun the journey towards portraying this story. Do you have existing skills or materials that you can employ? Perhaps embarking on this visualisation is the first step that you are grateful for taking. Ask the phoenix what the next stepping stone is to get you from where you currently are in this creative process to your destination. Does the phoenix deliver another egg or produce further images in the flames? Perhaps it speaks to you.

When you are ready, take a couple of deep breaths. Become aware of your surroundings and any sounds around you, wiggle your fingers and toes, open your eyes and jot down any inspiration you have received.

Return to this visualisation as often as you like.

Suggested therapeutic activity

Alternative translations

Choose a portion of your history that holds a distinctive emotion for you. It may be an event you've retold many times, or something you've never expressed despite it feeding its narrative into the heart of your being.

Have a go at telling it from a fresh perspective. Who else experienced this same event and how might they perceive it? If you enter their narrative, might you find a whole new slant on this memory that you hadn't previously considered, perhaps one that defuses some unpleasant charge? Consider the perspective of a healthcare professional, family member, onlooker, inanimate object or personified symptom. Journey into another's world and see how translating this part of your story into their language births new stories from the one you know so well.

If writing isn't your thing, there are other ways of recasting the past. Selina, who we heard from in previous chapters, suffers with complex PTSD. She knitted herself a trauma shawl, using colours that represent comfort, solace and positive memories from her childhood. Some of these recollections are extracted from the place of her trauma. By reclaiming them and now wrapping herself in this self-created celebration of survival, she gets to choose what memories she focuses on and how her story progresses.

Gathering the yarns of your life at a glance

- Stories are erupting from the world around you. Anything or anyone with a history, a perspective, or a potential future has its own story to tell.
- Consider what stories you can extract from mundane and unusual objects, conversations, memories and hopes.
- Do you have mementos from the past, saved remnants of a healthier you, or reminders of dreams abandoned. What stories do these hold?
- Stories needn't be literal, nor need they be fantastical. Any blend of realism and abstraction that works for you is fine.
- Stories needn't be formed from words – any craft can be employed to convey a story. It can be as simple or elaborate, as one-dimensional or multi-layered as you choose.
- How you live your own life story is a creative choice in itself. You get to choose the tone and style, if not the content. Be willing to change the genre of your own story or shift your focus into a parallel narrative that you are living with.
- Releasing your own story into the wild can give you a little space from its intensity.

Appendices

Creative directions

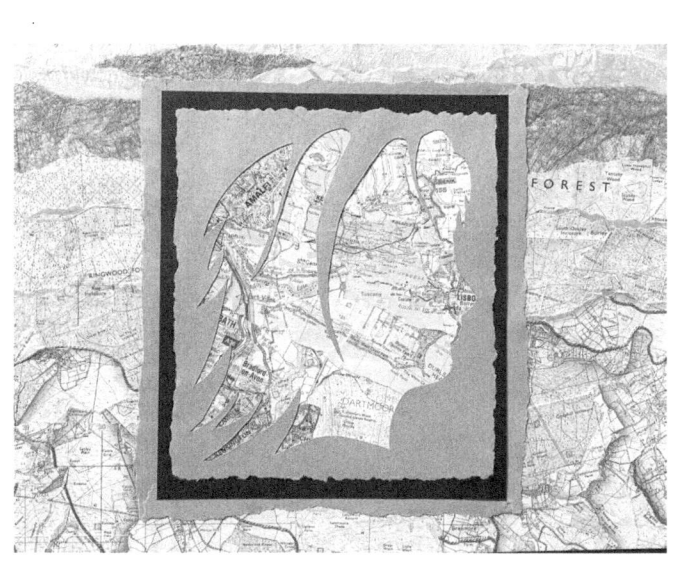

Appendix 1
Home-friendly arts and crafts

This list is by no means exhaustive. It is a selection of ideas for those of you looking to expand your creative repertoire. There are many more crafts that chronically ill people enjoy – fused glass and kiln-fired pottery, for example – but having access to a class or large and expensive equipment may be prohibitive. Many of the following suggestions can be enjoyed at home, on a hospital ward or in waiting rooms. The music category, rather than listing every available option, focuses predominantly on instruments that can be played sitting down or that aren't commonly considered.

Body art

Face and body painting
Hair styles and colouring
Make-up
Mendhi (temporary henna tattooing)
Nail art
Tattoo designs (can be printed on temporary tattoo transfer paper)

Culinary arts

Baking
Biscuit or cake decorating (using bought biscuits or cakes, if unable to bake)
Menus for virtual events and special days
Recipe design

Design

Architecture
Board games
Fantasy maps
Fantasy world building

Fashion design
Garden design
Interior design
Inventions and mechanical design
Tangrams
Web design

Drawing and paints

Acrylic paints and pens
Art journaling
Cartoons and graphic storytelling
Ceramic painting
Chalkboard art (a board painted with blackboard paint and set in a picture frame invites changeable art)
Chalk, charcoal and soft pastels
Colouring
Digital drawing and painting
Doodling
Dot painting
Encaustic art
Experimental mark-making (twigs, sponges, combs, scrunched up paper, erasers on the ends of pencils, etc., to transfer paint to a surface)
Gelli plate printing
Glass painting
Gouache paints
Hand lettering
Lino printing
Make-up art (eyeshadow, lipstick, etc., on paper)
Mandala drawing
Neurographic art (a specific form of attractive doodling designed to process emotions)
Oil pastels
Painting by numbers
Pebble and rock decorating (using paint, nail varnish, or pens)
Printing (potato-prints, leaves, cross-sections/undersides of mushrooms, printing blocks, a matchbox wrapped around with elastic bands, etc.)
Reverse colouring (random splodges of colour on a page that you look for patterns, images or shapes within, using a pen to draw these outlines. Reverse colouring books are available.)
Sgraffito
Stencilling (on paper, fabric, furniture, etc.)
Watercolour paints, pencils, pens, and/or crystals
Zentangles

Appendix 1

Modelling, mixed media and miscellaneous making

Air drying/hardening clay
Basketry
Beading
Book nook kits
Candles
Collages
Cosmetics and toiletries
Costumes
Diamond painting kits
Dioramas
Doll's house decoration
Glass painting
Home décor items
Jewellery
Kintsugi style visible mending
Masks (fantasy, Venetian, etc.)
Metal clay (small pieces can be fired using a butane torch, burning off the clay and leaving just the silver/ copper item)
Metal pressing/stamping kits
Model building
Mosaics
Plaster of paris moulding and casting
Polymer clay
Puppets
Pyrography
Resin art
Scratch art kits
Shadow boxes
Stained glass
Temporary mandalas, patterns or pictures (using a tray or shallow box, coloured sand, dried lentils, split peas, dry rice, etc.)
Upcycling
Wirework

Music

Composing
Digital music making
Drumming (bodhran, djembe, tabla, etc.)
Electric keyboard
Expressive movement (responding to music using whatever body parts you can)
Flute (traditional wooden style, held like a recorder)
Guitar
Jaw harp
Harmonica
Humming
Kalimba (a resin one is the quietest)
Lap harp
Recorder (treble recorders produce a deeper, more mellow sound than

descant)
Singing
Songwriting
Ukulele

Nature

Air plants
Bonsai trees
Corn dollies (materials or kits can be bought online) and St Brigid's crosses
Flower and leaf pressing
Flower arranging
Nature art (using found natural items)
Nature journaling (focusing on your garden, one tree, a patch of verge, a window view, or the weather through the year, etc.)
Pebble mosaics
Petal and leaf patterns and mandalas
Pot plants (including potted bulbs for spring flowers)
Raised beds and patio pots outside
Sand sculptures (using mouldable or dampened sand)
Seasonal wreaths
Tabletop zen sand garden kits
Terrarium or bottle garden
Willow craft/weaving
Windowsill salad and herb growing
Woodcarving

Papercraft

Book binding
Découpage
Die/digital cutting
Gift box and gift bag making
Greetings cards
Origami
Paper bead making
Paper-cut pictures
Paper dress-up characters (with changeable paper clothes attached via tabs)
Paper flowers
Paper making
Paper puppets
Paper sculptures
Paper theatre
Papier mâché
Picture collages
Pop-up books/cards
Quilling
Scrapbooking
Sticker books for adults
Zines

Appendix 1

Photography and film

Cyanotypes
Digital cartoons
Digital collaging
Film making
Photo editing
Photographing light, shadows, and movement
Photographing unusual angles or what you see from your bed/sofa
Shadow puppet films
Stop motion animation
Vlogging

Textiles, yarn and needlework

Amigurumi
Appliqué
Batik
Block printing
Boro
Crochet
Cross stitch
Dolls and soft toys, including clothes for them.
Dreamcatcher web weaving (the knotted technique can be used to simulate spiderwebs, insect wings, fairy wings and other decorative webs)
Dressmaking
Embroidery
Fabric wildlife (patterns for making stuffed fabric mushrooms, birds and other wildlife can be bought or you can design your own)
Friendship bracelets
God's eye weaving (also known as Bridie Eyes)
Kanzashi flowers (Japanese fabric flowers)
Knitting
Lacemaking (kits are available for the novice)
Lap loom weaving
Latch hooking
Loom knitting
Macramé (including micro macramé jewellery, keyrings, decorations, etc.)
Nalbinding (also known as needle binding)
Needle felting
Patchwork (machine sewn, crazy, or English paper piecing)
Pattern design
Quilting
Ribbon embroidery
Sashiko
Screen printing

Slow sewing (including creative mending)
Sock animals/monsters
Soft furnishings
Stitch diary (eg., each week for a year embroider a small image or word until you have filled a circle or other shape to frame, or a strip of fabric to wind around a stick or roll up as a textile scroll)
String art (also known as pin and thread art)
Stumpwork
Tapestry
Tatting
Textile collaging and artwork
Visible mending, using decorative or colourful stitches
Wet felting

Writing and words

Articles for websites and magazines
Blogging
Flash fiction and micro-fiction
Guided meditations/visualisations (written or recorded)
Journaling
Letter writing (to penpals, family members, or isolated members of society)
Memoire writing or recording
Non-fiction essays/books
Novels/novellas
Oral storytelling
Poetry (freeform, haikus, limericks, concrete poetry, ekphrastic poetry, acrostics, black out poetry, etc.)
Prose vignettes
Re-telling traditional myths, legends or fairy tales
Reviews of books and other products
Short stories
Treasure hunts and word puzzles for others

Appendix 2
Charity and kindness projects

A web search for any of the following should bring up all the information you will need, to get involved.

Cards and letter writing

Card-making Circle accepts handmade cards for them to sell to raise money for charities.
Cards for Bravery distribute handmade cards to hospitalised or seriously ill children.
The Christmas Card Project, run by Action for ME, accepts homemade or bought and filled out cards to ease the seasonal loneliness of participating members with ME.
Chronically Creative Cards for ME/CFS was created for patients with severe ME but accommodates any chronic illness. Sign up to be a giver or receiver, or both.
Festive Friends, in partnership with Contact the Elderly, invite you to send Christmas cards for them to forward on.
Health Story Collaborative shares and honours real life health stories told in any creative medium (no more than 1500 words, if written).
The World Needs More Love Letters encourages you to handwrite and post kind letters to people on their list of recipients in need around the world.
Post Pals encourages you to send cards, letters, emails, and gifts if you like, to seriously ill children and their siblings. Their Facebook group also holds annual auctions of donated handmade items to raise funds.
The Warrior Card Swap is a monthly global event purely for illness warriors to encourage each other by sending and receiving cards.
Write for Rights, run every winter by Amnesty International, shares a list of oppressed people and prisoners of conscience to send cards of support to.

Crochet and knitting

Blankets for the Homeless – Co Durham Pod (a Facebook group) requires volunteers anywhere to either knit or crochet squares, or sew them together into completed blankets.

The Buddy Bag Foundation distributes backpacks filled with useful and comforting items for children in emergency care. They include knitted teddies donated by the public.

Cats Protection and other animal rescue centres often require knitted blankets for animals in their care.

Charity Crafters is a Facebook group where you can sell your handmade items and donate the proceeds to charities of your choice.

Charity Squares Chat Group is a Facebook group offering knitting, crochet and loom patterns as well as suggestions for places to send your finished squares to for them to be included in blankets for those in need.

Christmas Angels are knitted by volunteers, and sent to participating members of Action for ME. The simple pattern is supplied online.

Commit to Knit runs an appeal every autumn for knitted and crocheted hats for the homeless.

Crochet a Granny Square is a Facebook group that collects squares crocheted by group members and donated by post to make into blankets for charities.

Easter Chick Appeal is an annual appeal in which thousands of knitted and crocheted chicks and bunnies (patterns supplied online) are filled with crème eggs and sold to raise money for Francis House Children's Hospice.

The Gift of Warmth is a Facebook group that appeals for knitted or crocheted baby clothes, teddies, completed blankets and squares to contribute to blankets.

Handmade with Love for Preemies UK welcome knitted or crocheted blankets, bonding squares, cannula mitts, cardigans, ear savers and hats (including traffic light hats).

Hookers and Clickers Do It For Charity work with local, national and international charities, with the aim to make the world better one knitted or crocheted stitch at a time.

Appendix 2

Knit A Square accept crocheted and knitted squares for them to make into blankets for vulnerable children and orphans in South Africa.

Knit for Peace supply a list of groups around the country requiring knitted donations, as well as supplying patterns and accepting items themselves to send around the world.

Knit for Sands require knitted or crocheted white blankets to include in their memory boxes for bereaved parents.

Knitted Knockers are knitted or crocheted prosthetic breasts, made by volunteers, for women who have undergone a mastectomy or lumpectomy.

The Mother Bear Project invites you to knit or crochet teddies for children affected by HIV/AIDS in emerging nations.

Octopus for a Preemie encourages you to crochet an octopus with tentacles that resemble umbilical cords, to be distributed to a neonatal ward where new-borns find them comforting to grip.

Petals of Gratitude (UK) is a Facebook group for people who would like to crochet flowers for cancer patients to give to their healthcare workers as a token of appreciation.

Random Acts of Crochet Kindness UK is a Facebook group that encourages members to crochet items to leave, along with an explanatory note, in public places for anyone to take.

Sanddancer Scarves for the Homeless is a Facebook group that appeals for knitted or crocheted scarf donations.

Sew Knit Crochet for the NHS and Charities is a Facebook group that welcomes appeals from different charities and works as a hub for those who like to donate their work.

Stitches of Support, organised by The Nightingale Cancer Support Centre, invites knitters and crocheters to contribute squares that will be joined together into blankets for people with cancer. Example patterns are provided online.

Trauma Teddies and Bobby Buddies are simple knitted teddies handed out to traumatised children. Contact any police/fire station or A&E department to see if they are participating. For the patterns, type Trauma Teddies or Bobby Buddies into a search engine.

Twiddle muffs and **fidget teddies** are often required by hospitals and care homes for autistic patients and those suffering with dementia. Patterns can be found online.

Ukraine Uzhhorod hospital Donations help knit crochet craft group is a British Facebook group that takes clothes, toys and blankets to Ukraine. They also accept squares for making up into blankets.

United By Wool – Helping Those in Need is a friendly Facebook group for knitters and crocheters creating items for charities and good causes. They share tips and patterns.

The Warm Baby Project invites you to knit baby items and to take part in their mystery knits.

Woolly Hugs have ongoing projects to contribute to, including comfort blankets for seriously ill children, refugee families, bereaved parents and women undergoing cancer treatment. They also encourage volunteers to crochet or knit random acts of kindness hearts.

The Yarny Army is a knitting group that makes items for use within NHS healthcare settings. Patterns are provided online and items can be sent from afar.

Sewing

The Craftivist Collective suggests gentle acts of activism, usually via stitched projects. These are detailed on their website and can be bought as kits.

Dress a Girl Around the World send handmade dresses and shorts, made by volunteers, to children living in poverty. Despite its name, clothes are sent to boys as well.

Fidget mats or **sensory quilts** are calming for those with dementia and autism. Care homes and hospitals are often in need of them. Patterns and ideas can be found online.

Little Dresses for Africa – UK is a Facebook group that delivers simple dresses and shorts, made by volunteers, to vulnerable boys and girls in Africa.

Love Quilts invites you to cross stitch designs to be included in bespoke quilts for seriously ill children. Details can be found on their website.

Making for Charity request items to assist those receiving cancer treatment, including syringe driver/drainage bottle bags, comfort pack bags, personal belongings bags and connection hearts.

Project Linus UK aims to provide comfort to sick, disabled and disadvantaged children through patchwork blankets.

Sewing for Charity is a Facebook group that encourages you to make, among other items, washable sanitary pads for areas affected by disasters around the world.

Sew Knit Crochet for the NHS and Charities is a Facebook group that welcomes appeals from different charities and works as a hub for those who like to donate their work.

Various arts and crafts

The Art for Charity Collective holds auctions selling donated artwork to raise funds for charities.

A Space Between connects with hospitals and communities to provide flexible, adaptable spaces of creative calm. They use colouring-in designs that are donated by artists and creatives from all walks of life.

Bake4MECFS raises money for ME charities through online baking competitions open to anyone for the cost of a donation. If you are unable to bake your entry, they can assign a collaborative baker to bring your design to life on your behalf.

Loose Ends finishes projects that people are unable to complete due to illness, disability or death. These are then returned to the family or intended recipient. You can apply to have a project finished on your behalf or to become a volunteer crafter, using your skill (mostly textiles and yarn work but also basketry) to complete what another has begun.

The Resonance Project is appealing for singers and musicians to record themselves contributing to a musical score to be used on a documentary raising awareness of invisible illnesses.

The (Secret) Toy Society encourages people to leave handcrafted toys, along with a note, where strangers can find them and take them home.

Appendix 3
Online resources

The internet is far too vast a place for me to list all the creative resources to be found there. What follows is merely a selection of pleasurable haunts and useful avenues. Facebook, alone, abounds with groups for all kinds of artists, crafters and appreciators, so I have limited that section to creativity groups specifically for chronically ill members.

Art and craft courses, talks, workshops and competitions

Arvon is a charity that offers online writing courses, classes and talks (some free of charge) through their Arvon at Home option.
Craftsy provides tutorials and online classes, from baking and gardening to quilting and woodworking.
Creative Bug offers thousands of art and craft video lessons as well as downloadable patterns and recipes.
CRIPtic Arts aims to ignite disabled excellence across the arts. They offer events, including online workshops for disabled writers, and have collaborated with Spread the Word to form **CRIPtic x Spread the Word Salons** which are bi-monthly online workshops and readings for deaf and disabled writers.
The Disabled Poets Prize is an annual competition open to anyone over 18, living in the UK, who identifies as deaf or disabled.
Domestika is an online community for creatives, offering many and varied courses.
London Drawing Group offers online lectures and art classes with payment by donation only.
Moving Mountains brings together, via anthologies and online workshops,

nature writing and those who live with chronic illness or physical disability.
Skillshare supplies thousands of hands-on creative classes via the internet.
Virtual Village Hall offers free online activities with sessions led by tutors.
Writers HQ has online writing classes and courses with bursaries for some applications.

Creative inspiration

Disability Arts Online shares disability arts and culture with the world. It includes a magazine, directory, projects and events.

Google Arts and Culture is available via either its website or app. Over 2000 museums and archives are featured, many of which offer virtual exhibits and tours, including Frida Kahlo's Blue House and the Getty Museum.

Health Story Collaborative shares and honours real life health stories told in any creative medium.

Museum of International Folk Art has some online exhibitions as well as resources for DIY folk art.

The Nightstand Collective shares submitted photographs of the bedside tables of those with chronic illness.

Online Art & Craft Club, held monthly by Bristol Libraries, is for anyone anywhere to share what they've been working on.

Pillow Crafters is a subgroup of Pillow Writers. Meet via video call for therapeutic crafting (no obligation to be creating) while chatting.

Pillow Writers is an online writing group for those with ME/CFS or Long Covid. They meet via video call to share short-form writing every week and to share long-form writing every other week.

Pinterest allows you to search for anything, see what inspiration you uncover, and save what you like to your own boards of ideas, as well as following others'.

Ravelry is a crochet and knitting pattern database. Many of the patterns are free.

Resting Up Collective is a group of chronically ill and disabled people practising slowness to create and interrupt expectations on the body. It is open to all. Subscribe for full access to the website and zine.

Sick is a magazine by chronically ill and disabled people, seeking to elevate their voices. It welcomes submissions in the form of visual art, poetry, essays, interviews and more.

Spoonie Press is a publisher, community, and disability advocate featuring an online magazine and hardcopy journal made for and by creative disabled, chronically ill, and neurodiverse people. Submissions are welcomed.

Still Ill Ok is an online arts hub for chronically ill artists and accessibility activists. It includes a zine that is open to submissions.

Stitchlinks is a global support network for those who enjoy the therapeutic effects of crafts. Free knitting patterns can be found on the site.

Surviving Severe ME is a website by the author Claire Wade that includes suggestions and links for creating virtual holidays.

This is Colossal is an online archive of thousands of articles featuring the visual arts.

The Weaving Loom is an online guide to all kinds of lap loom weaving, including lessons and making a cardboard loom.

Wishbone Words is an online magazine for chronically ill writers and artists. It is a safe, supportive, and understanding platform.

Facebook communities for chronically ill creatives

Chronic Creatives is an ever-growing group for people who are creative but have to work around chronic illness(es). There are subsidiary groups run by members of Chronic Creatives for specific interests, such as gardening, photography, and writing.

Chronic Market is a US-based platform for creatives who suffer from ME/CFS. As well as selling handmade items Chronic Market hosts virtual gatherings for people around the world, including healthy allies.

Conscious Crafties is a worldwide selling site and community for hand-crafters and artists who live with chronic illness or disabilities, or who care for a loved one.

Crafters With Chronic Illness is a small, friendly group that also welcomes those who support someone with chronic illness.

Customize My Mobility Aid: The Comeback encourages members to personalise their mobility aids. Members share photos of their decorated aids along with creative tips.

Long Covid Choir and **Long Covid Kids Choir** are held weekly online for breathing exercises, singing (on mute if you like) and optional chat. Drop in and out whenever you like.

Long Covid and ME/CFS Healing Through Creativity encourages creativity to process, heal and produce beauty from a horrible situation.

Pillow Writers has a Facebook group for those with ME/CFS or Long Covid that you can engage with whether or not you attend the online writing group.

Support for ill and disabled artists

Authors with Disabilities and Chronic Illnesses (ADCI) offers support and guidance for disabled authors, including those living with chronic illness. It is available to members of the Society of Authors.

Chronically Ill Artists Network works nationally to provide support, opportunities, information and advocacy for chronically ill disabled artists who currently work, want to work, or have previously worked in the arts.

Ciadish is a magazine for chronically ill and disabled writers and the readers who love their books. It includes book reviews, interviews, events, and more.

Outside In is a charity for artists facing barriers due to health, disability, social circumstance or isolation.

Appendix 4
Metaphors and imagery to explore

When we sharpen our attention, stories and themes reveal themselves all around. The suggestions that follow, sourced from the arts, world mythologies and the natural world, lend themselves to the general experience of the chronically ill. Learn more about any that appeal to you and use them as immersions, creative launch pads or stepping stones on your creative way.

Stories and other writings

Alice in Wonderland drops away from the life she had taken for granted into a world where her body changes proportions, she is threatened with the loss of her head, and all usual logic has vanished. Even the resident cat has an unstable physical form.

Baba Yaga is a Slavic folk character who lives, some say, in a house on chicken legs that is never where it was last left and is a portal between the living world and the underworld. This abode could also be interpreted as the unpredictability of the physical body we live in. Baba Yaga herself is a terrifying old woman who insists on the performance of seemingly impossible tasks before delivering her gift of life-sustaining hearth-fire. This can represent the demands our conditions place on us and the gifts that lie beyond the struggles.

The Ballad of Thomas the Rhymer tells of a man led away to fairyland where time distorts for him while years pass in the everyday world.

Changeling tales abound in traditional literature and oral storytelling. When chronically ill, it can sometimes feel as if our true self has been stolen away and replaced.

The Gorilla in Your House is an allegory for living with chronic illness. It can be found online (details in the bibliography) and may well inspire your own take on it.

The Princess and the Pea is a fairy tale that depicts a woman recognised as nobility by her awareness of the discomfort of a single pea under a pile of mattresses. An apt tale for those with sensitive bodies.

Rapunzel may not be ill or disabled but the main character of this fairy tale is shut away, alone and out of easy reach in her door-less room at the top of a tower.

Rip van Winkle, written by Irving Washington, is a short story about a man who sleeps for twenty years, missing historical events.

Rumpelstiltskin may feel relevant to those with an un-named illness or delayed diagnosis. The naming of something changes the power balance, and we also have the motif of spinning gold from straw in this classic folktale.

Selkies feature in folk stories predominantly of Celtic and Norse origin. They are seals who have shed their animal skin to take the form of a human while on land. If their sealskin is hidden from them, preventing them from returning to their true state, they ail and pine for their original existence. Aspects of these tales always remind me of living in an ill state that doesn't feel aligned with my natural spirit.

The Sleeping Beauty is a classic fairy tale, perfect for re-imagining under the gaze of illness.

The Sleeping Hero/The King in the Mountain is a motif in Arthurian legend as well as myths and folktales around the world. The King or hero will awake when he is needed to save his country. This moment is sometimes said to be presaged by the dying out of birds, which connects with the concept of the canary in the coal mine.

The Tortoise and the Hare is a classic Aesop's fable teaching the importance of taking things slowly and steadily.

The Ugly Duckling speaks of finally finding our tribe and of accepting ourselves when we don't fit in with what is considered normal.

The Wounded/Fisher King is part of the Arthurian legend. Its leaning towards injury and illness being the result of dubious morality makes it prime material for subversion and revisioning.

Appendix 4

Visual imagery

Canary in a Coal Mine is an image that represents early warning signs of danger. Some feel that illness can shine a light on potential changes that could improve life in general for all members of society.

Labyrinths are a specific form of maze that wind around in one circuitous path before delivering you at the centre. They represent wholeness through the spiralling journey to the core of ourselves before returning out into the world again.

Magic carpets takes us magically away. Where can you creatively travel with a magic carpet to work with?

Mazes represent the thwarted intentions and uncertain path through chronic illness, but also the destination at the centre of ourselves and the easier path thereon.

Mermaids in wheelchairs feature in the artwork of Ernie Fuglevand. An internet search will reveal his representations of disability that doesn't sit down meekly.

Mosaics are a powerful symbol of the broken and discarded becoming something new. Fragments join together to create something greater than the sum of its parts.

Mud Maid is a prone woman made from the landscape at The Lost Gardens of Heligan in Cornwall. She is a part of the environment, at rest with her stillness. Images of her lying down throughout the seasons can be found online.

Phoenix images remind us of the power to rise from the ashes of what has been burnt away. We may rise in the resurrected image of our past self or as someone different.

Reclining Buddha statues represent the Buddha during his last illness before his death. Death can be viewed as symbolic as well as literal.

Resting Buddha statues depict the Buddha sitting upright but relaxing peacefully with his head resting on his hands.

Spirals are symbols of creativity, natural energy and the spiralling path through life as we travel around, re-experiencing things in new ways and with wider perspective. Anti-clockwise spirals represent decrease and letting go, while clockwise spirals represent increase and growth.

Tarot cards provide plenty of interesting imagery to consider. The Hermit may feel relevant to those who are isolated by long-term illness, while The Hanged Man signifies a pause during which things are seen from a new perspective and is reminiscent of the image of Odin hanging from the world tree. Meanwhile, The Tower represents everything crashing down around you to make way for a better future, and The Star speaks of bright hope after difficult times.

Deities

Aengus/Angus is a Celtic god of poetic inspiration and sweet dreams, having had a dream that lasted over a year in which he searched for his true love. In the eponymous song, Dream Angus is said to 'hirple', meaning limp or hobble. His breath holds the power of resurrection, albeit sometimes a temporary reprieve.

Ebistu is a Japanese god born without bones and rejected by his parents. Adopted by a kinder father, he grows a skeleton but retains some disability and lives a merry, mirthful life. He shares joy and luck with all, regardless of circumstance.

Hephaestus is a Greek god who used the taunts he received due to his limp as a catalyst for his art.

Icarus, in Greek mythology, was instructed to fly neither too low towards the sea nor too high towards the sun, teaching us about finding our most sustainable path.

Inanna, later known by the Babylonians as Ishtar, was a Sumerian goddess who had to pass through seven gates during her descent to the underworld, at each gate letting go of more of her upperworld identity. She mirrors the many sacrifices and losses that chronic illness can bring with it.

Kali is the Hindu goddess of destruction and creation, time and change. In the past, I have imagined my illness as Kali-Ma (Mother Kali) stamping on the battlefield of my body before nurturing new growth.

Appendix 4

Odin is removed from daily life for nine days when hung from Ygdrassil, the world tree, in Norse mythology. In doing this he learns the secrets of the runes (the ancient Nordic alphabet). The more recent concept of Odinsleep is created by Marvel for their depictions of Odin in their comics. It is his periodic need for deep rest to recharge his magical force.

Persephone is lost to the underworld for six months of every year. While she resides there her mother, the Greek earth goddess Demeter, mourns her loss and winter reigns. When Persephone returns to spend time with her mother, the earth flourishes and blooms. This is a powerful myth to represent the fluctuating nature of chronic illness and reminds us that we still hold value even in our absence from the visible world.

Nature

Beetles have long larval stages before they become visible above ground as beetles. One type of wood boring beetle takes 51 years to emerge from its larval stage. Stag beetles spend between three to seven years in larval form, residing up to half a metre underground or in dead wood, before emerging to live for just a few weeks in the form that we see. This is a reminder of hidden and dormant aspects of nature being as much a part of life as the visibly active stages.

Deciduous trees and perennial plants are stripped to their skeletons or diminished to their roots over winter, but they return each year after a period of dormancy.

Hibernating animals hold obvious imagery for those of us with hypersomnolence or tucked away in our homes.

Nests and burrows are places of comfort and safety and a way to re-vision the feeling of being imprisoned when housebound.

Pupae and cocoons of any species. Caterpillars securing themselves away to transform into butterflies have become something of a trope but are still a powerful analogy for those feeling their old self disintegrate.

Seeds, including pips, acorns, etc., all hold great potential in their tiny dormant forms. They fall to the ground where they gestate in the darkness, sometimes for years, before reaching up to the light again.

Snakes, due to regularly shedding their skin, remind us of the value of letting go of old forms of ourselves, as well as symbolising both recurring cycles and healing. As such, snakes wrapped around a staff have come to represent medicine via the Rod of Aesculapius (one snake) and the Caduceus (two snakes).

Bibliography

Books

Altan, Ahmet. *I Will Never See the World Again*. Granta Books, 2019.

Burrus, Christina. *Frida Kahlo: 'I Paint My Reality'*. Thames and Hudson Ltd, 2008.

Cameron, Julia. *The Right to Write: An Invitation and Initiation into the Writing Life*. Hay House, UK, 2017.

Carr, Susan. *Portrait Therapy: Resolving Self-Identity Disruption in Clients with Life-Threatening and Chronic Illnesses*. Jessica Kingsley Publishers, 2017.

Corkill, Betsan. *Knit for Health and Wellness: How to knit a flexible mind and more…* FlatBear Publishing, 2014.

Fancourt, Daisy. *Arts in Health: Designing and researching interventions*. Oxford University Press, 2017.

Fox, John. *Poetic Medicine*. Penguin Publishing Group, 1997.

Frank, Arthur. *The Wounded Storyteller*. University of Chicago Press, 2013.

Frankl, Viktor E. *Man's Search for Meaning: The classic tribute to hope from the Holocaust*. Ebury Digital, 2013.

Graham-Pole, John. *Illness and the Art of Creative Self-expression*. New Harbinger Publications, 2000.

Hunter, Clare. *Threads of Life: A History of the World Through the Eye of a Needle*. Sceptre, 2020.

Kaimal, Girija. *The Expressive Instinct: How Imagination and Creative Works Help Us Survive and Thrive*. Oxford University Press, 2022.

Kaufman, Scott Barry, and Gregoire, Carolyn. *Wired to Create*. Ebury Digital, 2016.

Kleon, Austin. *Steal Like an Artist*. Workman, 2012.

Lehrer, Riva. *Golem Girl: A Memoir*. Virago, 2021.

Lowe, Sarah M and Fuentes, Carlos. *The Diary of Frida Kahlo: An Intimate

Self-Portrait. Abrams in association with La Vaca Independiente, 2006.

Magsamen, Susan and Ross, Ivy. *Your Brain On Art – How the Arts Transform Us.* Canongate Books Ltd, 2023.

Maistre, de Xavier. *A Journey Around My Room.* www.gutenberg.org/ebooks/62519.

Perillo, Lucy. *I've Heard the Vultures Singing: Field Notes on Poetry, Illness and More.* Trinity University Press, US, 2007.

Saltz, Jerry. *How To Be an Artist.* Ilex Press, 2020.

Sandblom, Philip. *Creativity and Disease.* Marion Boyars, 7th edition, 1995.

Stuart-Smith, Sue. *The Well Gardened Mind – Rediscovering Nature in the Modern World.* William Collins, 2020.

Woolf, Virginia and Bell, Quentin. *Selected Diaries: Virginia Woolf.* Vintage Classics, 2008.

Zausner, Tobi. *When Walls Become Doorways: Creativity and the Transforming Illness.* Kindle edition, 2016.

Online articles and research papers

Arruda MALB, Garcia MA, Garcia JBS. Evaluation of the Effects of Music and Poetry in Oncologic Pain Relief: A Randomized Clinical Trial. *J Palliat Med* 2016; 19(9): 943-948. DOI: 10.1089/jpm.2015.0528

Berlinson, Lauren. Take A Line for a Lie-Down: A Conversation with Paula Knight. The Big Draw. https://thebigdraw.org/take-a-line-for-a-lie-down-a-conversation-with-paula-knight. 2022 (Accessed 24 November 2024)

Cetinkaya F. The effects of listening to music on postoperative nausea and vomiting. *Complement Ther Clin Pract* 2019; 35: 278-283. DOI: 10.1016/j.ctcp.2019.03.003

Conrad C. Music for Healing: from magic to medicine. *Lancet* 2010; 376(9757): 1980-1981.

Dadka B Anisi E, Mozaffari N, Amani F, Pourghasemian M. Effect of Music Therapy with Periorbital Massage on Chemotherapy-Induced Nausea and Vomiting In Gastrointestinal Cancer: A Randomized Controlled Trial. *J Caring Sci* 2019; 8(3): 165-171. DOI: 10.15171/jcs.2019.024

Bibliography

Da Ros G. That's Why They Don't Believe You, You Don't Look Sick!: Fictional Representations of ME/CFS. 26 January, 3 March, 8 April 2022. www.meaction.net/author/giada/ (Accessed 24 November 2024)

Dufrene PM. Utilizing The Arts for Healing From A Native American Perspective: Implications For Creative Arts Therapies. 1998 www.semanticscholar.org/paper/UTILIZING-THE-ARTS-FOR-HEALING-FROM-A-NATIVE-FOR-Dufrene/95f57896309c262bb062a8f3c03339b7fa394f34 (Accessed 24 November 2024)

Duda, Sue. 'I Grieved the Loss of My Identity as a Potter.' (craftforhealth.typepad.com, 2011.)

Fabella, Mara. 'The T'nalak of the Tboli.' (narrastudio.com)

Gutierrez, Katie. 'The Best Keys for Relaxation.' (brightstarmusical.com, 2022.)

Health Foundation, The. 'The Power of Storytelling.' (health.org.uk, 2016.)

Hillenbrand, Laura. 'A Sudden Illness: How My Life Changed.' *The New Yorker*, 2003.

Househam AM, Peterson CT, Mills PJ, Chopra D. The Effects of Stress and Meditation on the Immune System, Human Microbiota, and Epigenetics. *Adv Mind Body Med* 2017; 31(4): 10-25.

Jordan J. 'Susana Clarke: "I was cut off from the world, bound in one place by illness."' *The Guardian* 12 September 2020. www.theguardian.com/books/2020/sep/12/susanna-clarke-i-was-cut-off-from-the-world-bound-in-one-place-by-illness (Accessed 24 November 2024)

Knit For Peace. 'The Health Benefits of Knitting.' (knitforpeace.org.uk/wp-content/uploads/2017/05/The-Health-Benefits-of-Knitting-Preview.pdf)

Lee, Tom. 'The Benefits of Chronic Illness' (theparisreview.org, 2019.)

Leggett, Hadley. '"Cyclic Sighing" Can Help Breathe Away Anxiety' (scopeblog.stanford.edu, 2023.)

Mascarelli, Amanda. 'Might Crafts Such as Knitting Offer Long-term Health Benefits?" *The Washington Post*, 2014.

McGuire KMB. Autonomic Effects of Expressive Writing in Individuals with Elevated Blood Pressure. *Journal of Health Psychology* 2005; 10(2): 197-209. DOI: 10.1177/1359105305049767

Miserandino, Christine. 'The Spoon Theory.' (butyoudontlooksick.com)

Plotner, Jordan. 'The Resonance Project.' (jordanplotner.com, 2019.)

Powell, Esta. 'Catharsis in Psychology and Beyond: A Historic Overview.' (primal-page.com)

Riley J, Corkhill B, Morris C. The Benefits of Knitting for Personal and Social Wellbeing in Adulthood: Findings from an International Survey. *British Journal of Occupational Therapy* 2013; 76(2): .
DOI: 10.4276/030802213X13603244419077

Standford SPARQ. 'Caring Letters Prevent Suicide.' (sparq.stanford.edu)

Stuckey HL, Nobel J. The connection between art, healing, and public health: a review of current literature. *Am J Public Health* 2010; 100(2): 254-263.

'The Gorilla In Your House.' (batsgirl.blogspot.com. 2008.)

University Hospitals, The Science of Health. 'The Science Behind Kindness and How It Benefits Your Health.' (uhhospitals.org. 2020.)

Vogin, Gary D. 'Humming May Help Sinuses Stay Healthy: Increases Airflow, Which May Fight Sinus Infections.' (WebMD, 2002.)

Weitzberg E, Lundberg JON. Humming Greatly Increases Nasal Nitric Oxide. *Am J Respir Crit Care Med* 2002; 166(2): 144-145.
DOI: 10.1164/rccm.200202-138BC

Welsh NHS Confederation. 'Arts, health and wellbeing.' (nhsconfed.org, 2018.)

Williams, Holly. 'The Unseen Masterpieces of Frida Kahlo.' (bbc.com/culture, 2021.)

Podcasts and radio programmes

Creative Fuel
Creative Pep Talk
Hidden Brain
Invisible Not Broken – Chronic Illness Podcast Network
Post-Exertional Mayonnaise
Sketches: Stories of art and people (BBC Radio 4, 2021.)
Start With This

Television programmes and YouTube videos

Craftivism: Making A Difference. (BBC, 2021.)

Fruity Knitting. 'Ergonomics of Knitting – Carson Demers.' (YouTube, 2017 and 2020.)

Grayson's Art Club. (Channel 4, 2021.)

Acknowledgments

Crafting a Path Through Illness wouldn't have been written without input from others. Thank you to La Vaca Independiente for permission to reproduce extracts from The Diary of Frida Kahlo; to everyone who was happy for me to share their words and experiences; and to all whose creativity and perspectives have informed this book. It feels fitting to take a moment here to remember S-J, who was still alive when I wrote about her in Chapter 9. S-J was particularly supportive of my endeavours to send this book out into the wild. She lives on in the warm memories many hold of her.

Winning a free manuscript assessment through Arvon and The Literary Consultancy gave me the opportunity to find out how my work may be received and boosted my confidence in sending it out to seek a publisher. Speaking of which, Hammersmith Books has quite literally brought my dream to life. Huge appreciation to Georgina Bentliff for wholeheartedly embracing my offering, and Madeline Meckiffe for the cover design that allows my origami butterflies to fly out into the world.

Special thanks to Selina L. Wilkinson for planting the seed that my creative approach to living with unremitting illness is something others would benefit from reading about, and watering that seed with continued belief in my abilities; Victoria Flute for founding Chronic Creatives, the Facebook group that re-awakened my creativity and connected me with so many others in similar situations; Andy McLellan for the fresh translation of Issa's "O Snail" haiku (as so often, you were there exactly when needed!); and Anna Wood for enthusiastic support and hosting a virtual getaway to Glasgow when I was in need of distraction from thinking about editing.

Family is the fertile soil from which the patterns of my branches grow. I wholly appreciate the cheerleading and practical help, notably: Mum for encouraging and enabling my creative pursuits right from the beginning, believing that my writing should be read far and wide, contributing constructive criticism on an early draft, and always being there to bounce thoughts and ideas off; Jack for regular therapeutic massages; Leela for appreciation and admiration of whatever I'm able to do (you inherited my condition, yes, but also more creativity than you give yourself credit for so remember to admire yourself, too!); and Dom for looking after everything, including me, while urging me to use my crumbs of energy to feed whatever brings creative comfort, as well as offering helpful feedback whenever asked (thank you, Dom, for turning your wild spirit towards our home-grown pleasures and adventures).

And finally, my gratitude to my body for allowing me to write this book before descending into deeper symptoms.

Index

Abiligrip 184
acceptance and acknowledgement (of circumstances) 4, 17, 21, 62, 110, 122, 173, 176, 252
accessible creativity 181–209
accommodation 16, 164, 165, 172–173
acknowledgement and acceptance (of circumstances) 4, 17, 21, 62, 110, 122, 173, 176, 252
acrylic paint 199, 204
activism and crafts (craftivism) 83–84
adrenaline 58, 59, 144, 151, 169
Aengus (Angus) 328
affirmation 236
 of our strengths 21
agency (personal) 63, 64, 79, 300
aids/equipment/tools 22, 181–209
alarm calls/warning signs 135, 143
Alice in Wonderland 325
Alice in Wonderland syndrome 27
ally, creativity as 11–12
aloneness (solitude and loneliness) 91–92, 95, 98, 101
Altan, Ahmet 249
altar, creating an 275–276
Alter, Adam 155
altruism 86
amulet, inner 262

amygdala 54, 58, 127, 278
anagram-solving 293
ancient civilisations 37–43
Andy (ill person) 33, 178, 225
Angus (Aengus) 328
Anna (ill person) 95–96, 189–190
Anna B (ill person) 212, 218–219
Anna M (ill person) 218
anxiety 57–58
aphasia 267
appliqué 195–196
Arabia, 11th century 39
Aristotle 37, 38, 272
arm (one) out of action 189
art and craft 23–27, 37–43
 aids/equipment/tools 22, 181–209
 craft kits 12–13, 83, 196–197, 222, 227
 expressive 80
 historical perspectives 23–27, 37–43
 home-friendly 309
 imposter feeling 97–98
 life as work of art 15–16
 limited sessions 250
 neuroplasticity and 45–46
 online resources *see* online
 physical conditions and 45–52
 size (of product) 164–166

tensions in 127–133
various sources 318–319
art and craft therapy, official emergence 41
Art for Charity Collective 319
artists (ill and disabled) 23–34
   historical/well-known 23–30, 34
   support 324
Arvon 321
Asclepius, temples to 37
Atwood, Margaret 288
Aurelius, Marcus 70, 76
Authors with Disabilities and Chronic Illnesses (ADCI) 324
awareness of self 130, 236

Baba Yaga 325
Bake4MECFS 319
Ballad of Thomas the Rhymer 325
beading 197
Beckett (ill person) 113
bed, confined/bound to (bedbound) 199, 271
   author 2, 72, 223, 227, 273
beetles 329
being vs doing 70
birds 85
blackout poetry 203
Blankets for the Homeless – Co Durham Pod 316
blogs 74
Bobby Buddies 87, 317
body
   cycle, paying attention to 145
   listening to language of 165
   posture 137–138
   warning signs/alarm calls 135, 143, 149
body art 309
body of creativity 13–14
body scan 141

Bolles, Kyrianna 34
Bondaweb 196
book(s)
   holding open 184–185
   kindness bookmarks 87
borrowing from others (other persons) 285–289
brain
   amygdala 54, 58, 127, 278
   cognitive impairment/deficit 11, 46, 190
   foggy 32, 83, 176, 182, 190, 202, 205, 267, 269, 279
   HPA (hypothalamus-pituitary-adrenal) axis 52, 58
   neuroplasticity 45–46, 49
   neurotransmitters 55, 57, 129
   physical conditions and 45, 46, 49
   stress and 140
breaks *see* stopping
breathing, cyclic 140–141
Brewster, Dr Annie 99
Buddhism
   Buddha statues 327
   Tibetan 56
Buddy Bag Foundation 316
burrows 329
butterflies
   caterpillars transforming into 329
   origami 116–117

calmness and health 53–66
cameras and film/photography 2, 204–205, 312
canary in a coal mine 327
card(s) 315
   postcards from another reality 282–283
Card-making Circle 315
Cards for Bravery 315
carers, author's 73, 112

Index

Carr, M.D. 63
Carroll, Lewis 27
caterpillars transforming into butterflies 329
catharsis 37
   writing 37, 68
Cato (Roman) 38
Cats Protection 316
CFS *see* myalgic encephalomyelitis
chairs *see* sitting
Changeling 325
chants and incantations, medical 38, 42–43
Charity Crafters 316
charity and kindness projects 85, 315–319
Charity Squares Chat Group 316
children
   author's ME onset in childhood 2
   craft kits/art books 222
   parenthood and 73–74, 104
Chinese, ancient 38
choice, freedom of
   restricted 123
   too much (too many possibilities) 239–240, 251
Christina (ill person) 30–31
Christmas Angels 316
Christmas Card Project 315
Chronic Creatives 323
chronic fatigue syndrome *see* myalgic encephalomyelitis
chronic illness *see* illness
Chronic Market 323
Chronically Creative Cards for ME/CFS 315
Chronically Ill Artists Network 324
Chronically Inspired 33
Ciadish 324
circular needles 186
Clark, Susanna 28, 152, 221

classical music 49
clay 204
coastline paradox 273–274
cocoons 329
cognition
   illness cognition 62–63
   impairment/deficit 11, 46, 162, 190
collaborations, hidden 98
collage 51, 288
   borrowing from other people's work 288
   of life 20–21
colour wash 65–66
colouring 46–47
combinations and contradictions 291–297
comfort 227
   for others, knitting as 84–85
   see also discomfort
Commit to Knit 316
commitment certificate 170
communication (and connections/contact) 80–83, 91–105
community, power of 94–98
composers 29–30
confidence, creating 64–65
confusion and mess, starting with 173–175
connecting and connections (and communication/contact) 80–83, 91–105
Conscious Crafties 323
contact (and communication/connections) 80–83, 91–105
contentment 4
contradictions and combinations 291–297
Corrine (ill person) 71
cortisol 47, 54, 58
COVID-19 pandemic 52, 79–80, 103, 324

341

craft kits 12–13, 222
Crafters With Chronic Illness 323
craftivism 83–84
Craftivist Collective 83, 318
Craftsy 321
Creative Bug 321
Creative Pep Talk 81
creativity (basic references)
   accessible 181–209
   affirming *see* affirmation
   as ally 11–12
   body of (an exercise) 13–14
   creative life 9–14, 19, 115
   expanding our definition 212–214
   feedback loop 15–22
   health and 10–11
   healthcare and 35–43
   historical, viewpoints 37–43
   imagining it into existence 12–13
   legacy of 73–74
   life and *see* life
   making room for 119–125
   practice for *see* practice
   silent partner 214–215
   usefulness 84–85
   welcoming 235
CRIPtic Arts and CRIPtic x Spread the Word Salons 321
critic, inner (self-criticism) 171, 174, 178
crochet 129, 186–193, 316–319
   size considerations 164
   tools/equipment/aids 186–193
Crochet a Granny Square 316
cross-stitch 196–197
culinary arts 309
curiosity 21, 128, 129, 265, 295, 303
current (present) moment 55–56, 258
Customize My Mobility Aid: The Comeback 323–324
cut-out poetry 203

cutting, fabrics 194–195
cycles 223–226
   paying attention to body cycle 145
   sighing/breathing 140–141

dancing 63, 165
   mindful-based dance movement therapy 50
De Maistre, Xavier 277–278
dead ends 128, 166–167, 260
Deadly Knitshade 83
deciduous trees 329
decline something (need to) 120–121
decluttering 273
deities 276, 328–339
delegating 120–121
Demers, Carson 139
denial/denying (self-) 251, 254
depression 57–58
design(s) 309
   repetitive 240, 245
Dickinson, Emily 34
dining table 194–195
Disability Arts Online 322
Disabled Poets Prize 321
disappointments 128
   clinging to 294
   disappointing others 120–121
discomfort, conversation with 258
dislike and like 294, 296
disorder within a clearly delineated space 292, 293
diversional therapies 41
DK yarns 186
doing vs being 70
Domestika 321
doodling 46–47, 51, 133
dopamine 57, 129, 132
Dostoevsky, Fyodor 23
double knitting (DK) yarns 186
double-pointed needle 189

Index

drawing 46–47, 51, 310
   negative space 253
   pressure points 133
   tools/equipment/aids 198–201
dream journal 281–282
Dress a Girl Around the World 318
drumming 206
Duda, Sue 62
Duffy, Carol Ann 288
Dufy, Raoul 23

ear loops 206
Easter Chick Appeal 316
Ebistu 328
educating others 80–83
   see also learning
Ehlers-Danlos syndrome (EDS) 29–30, 82
elbows held close to body 138
Ellie (ill person) 32, 85
embroidery 196–197
EMDR (Eye Movement Desensitisation and Reprocessing) 61
Emma (ill person) 64
emotional difficulties 84
   re-directing 59–60
energy 135–159
   expenditure 124, 133, 151, 153, 155, 162, 188
   pushing and pacing see pacing; pushing
   reserves 91, 119, 145, 149, 158
   stopping up leaks 135–141
entertainment, therapeutic-grade 132
environment, maximising your 271–276
   see also space
equipment/tools/aids 22, 181–209
Ergonomic Knitter 139
errors and mistakes 175–177
Europe, music, historical perspectives 38–39

exertion see pushing
expectations 151, 181
   clinging to 294
experiences
   life see stories
   novel/new 111, 232, 241, 286
expressing oneself creatively 12, 158, 252, 253
expressive arts and crafts 80
expressive writing 48
Eye Movement Desensitisation and Reprocessing (EMDR) 61

fabrics see textiles
Facebook communities (for chronically ill creatives) 323–334
fallow times 211, 219, 226
fanciful imagination 277–283
feedback loop 15–22
felting 197–198
   needle 59, 198
Festive Friends 315
fiction-writing see novel-writing
fidget mats 318
fidget teddies 318
film/cameras/photography 2, 204–205, 312
fingers 183–185
   splints and yokes 184
First World War 41, 267
Fisher/Wounded King 327
flash fiction 109, 165, 281, 281
Flaubert, Gustave 27
flights of fancy 277–283
flow state 132–133, 145
flutes 206
foggy brain 32, 83, 176, 182, 190, 202, 205, 267, 269, 279
Fox, John 242
fragrance, following (exercise) 260–261
Frank, Arthur 299

Frankl, Viktor E 70–71, 76
freedom of choice *see* choice
fridge poetry set 203
Functionalhand 184

garden and gardening 49–51, 58, 85, 124, 207–208
Gift(s) 88, 103–104
   fallow-time 326
Gift of Warmth 316
glue sticks (fabrics) 195–196
goals (having) 171
   constructive sense of direction vs 75
   having none 129
gods *see* deities; religion
good practice 161–170
Google Arts and Culture 322
Google Docs 202
Gorilla in Your House 325
Goya, Francisco 24
graffiti knitting 83
Graham-Pole, John 40, 49, 58
Greece, ancient 37–38
grief and loss 61–62
grip aids 164, 184, 201
   pens/pencils/brushes 198, 201
groups (creativity) 30, 102
   in-person 102
   individuals' own words 30–34
   online/internet 93, 102, 178, 182
guided visualisations 303–305
gut microbiome 55

hand(s) (and their movements) 57, 130
   bilateral movements in EMDR 61
   rhythmic movements 37, 57
   shaky hands (tremors) 183, 200, 210
   tools/equipment/aids 183–185
handicrafts *see* art and craft
Handmade with Love for Preemies UK 316

health
   calmness 53–66
   purpose as predictor of healthy life 69–77
Health Story Collaborative 100, 315, 322
healthcare 35–66
   debris of 269–270
heat pads 138
help and support
   online *see* online
   for others 79–89
   for yourself 119–120
helping hand tool 183
Hephaestus 328
hibernating animals 329
Hill, Adrian 41
Hillenbrand, Laura 28
historical viewpoints 37–43
Holidays from Home 279
holistic health 40
honesty with yourself 121–122
Hookers and Clickers Do It For Charity 316
Horowitz, Anthony (author) 214
hospitals, art in 40, 49
housebound 3, 122, 244, 271, 280
   author 92, 231
   COVID-19 epidemic 79–80
HPA (hypothalamus-pituitary-adrenal) axis 52, 58
humming 50
humour 111, 268
hunger, paying attention to 136–137
Hunter, Clare 243
hypersensitivity of body 266
hypothalamus-pituitary-adrenal (HPA) axis 52, 58

Ibn Butlan 39
Icarus 328

Index

ice packs 138, 192
illness (chronic illness; physical
    conditions) 7–34, 91
  artists and *see* artists
  Facebook communities 323–334
  feeling larger than your illness
    67–105
  listening to voice of 265–270
  perfectionism as toxic partner of
    171–172
  restriction by *see* restrictions and
    limitations
  support *see* help and support
  wall 4
illness cognition 62
imagery 325–330
imagination 214, 279
  cultivating 215–217
  fanciful 277–283
  imagining creativity into existence
    12–13
imperfection, embracing 179
imposter feeling with art and craft
    97–98
Inanna 328
incantations, medical 38, 42–43
  see also singing
indoor gardening 208
inner artist 215
inner critic (self-criticism) 171, 174,
    178
inner self 257–263
insomnia 28, 181
inspiration (creative) 229–307
  meaning 234
  online resources 33, 322
integrating 80–83, 176
internal weather 245–246
internet *see* online
internet resources 321–324
Irish cottage knitting 189

Issa (Japanese poet) 225, 337

Jabeen (ill person) 173, 211
Jameson, Elizabeth 26, 82
Jo (ill person) 95
Jordan, Sarah-Louise 216
journalling
  dreams 281–282
  journal buddies 102–103

Kahlo, Frida 26, 34, 178, 271
Kaimal, Girija 46
Kali 328
kalimba 205–206
Karen (ill person) 32
Katie (ill person) 278–279
keyboards
  piano (electric) 205
  writing 201
Kiev (Kyiv Ukraine) 87
kindness and charity projects 85,
    315–319
King in the Mountain 326
Kiri (ill person) 30–31
kits 12–13, 83, 196–197, 222, 227
Klee, Paul 23, 200
Kleon, Austin 186
kneeler (gardening) 207–208
Knight, Paula 99, 200
Knit A Square 317
knit blockers 193
Knit for Peace 84, 317
Knit for Sands 317
Knitted Knockers 317
knitting 47, 55, 57–58, 186–193,
    316–319
  anxiety/depression and 57
  author's 19, 156
  as comfort for others 84–85
  errors 176
  graffiti knitting 83

345

individual's own words in a group 32–33
needles 66, 186–193
size considerations 164
tools/equipment/aids 186–193
Konrath, Dr Sara 80
Kyiv (Ukraine) 87

labyrinths 327
see also mazes
Lara (ill person) 164–165
laughter painting 29
learning
from others 286–289
pacing your 146–147
see also educating others
LED light-up crochet hooks and knitting needles 191
Lehrer, Riva (artist) 12
leisure *see* entertainment; play
letter-writing 314, 315
lever-action knitting 189
Libby (ill person) 272
life 9–14, 19, 115
collage of 20–21
past difficulties, art in responding to 259–260
sense of purpose/meaning 69–77
simplifying/uncomplicating 119–120
well lived 12, 77
as work of art 15–16
lifeline (in knitting) 190
light and lighting 136, 272
like and dislike 294, 296
listening *see* sounds; voice of illness
Little Dresses for Africa – UK 318
lived experiences *see* stories
London Drawing 321
loneliness (solitude and aloneness) 91–92, 95, 98, 101

Long Covid and ME/CFS Healing Through Creativity 324
Long Covid Choir 324
Long Covid Kids Choir 324
Loose Ends 319
loss
coming to terms with limitations and 63, 232, 252
grief and 61–62
love 71
Love Quilts 318

ma (white space - Japanese) 251, 253
machine sewing *see* sewing
magazine (UK - by author) 72–73, 150, 223
magic carpets 327
magnetic board words 203
magnifying glass 196
Mahler, Gustav 30
Mahli (ill person) 267
making a difference (to others) 79–89
Making for Charity 318–319
Makkin belt 189
Marion (ill person) 32, 214
Mary (ill person) 33
masterpieces, creating 178
Matisse, Henri 25
maximalism
continuum of minimalism and 21
maximising your environment 271–276
mazes 327
see also labyrinths
ME *see* myalgic encephalomyelitis
meaning (purpose), sense of 69–77
medicine
chants and incantations and 42–43
historical perspectives 28–29
trauma from 60
meditation 55–57

Index

Melissa (ill person) 129
memory and memories
   aids 182–183
   far-off 258
   reminiscing the past 258
Meniere's disease 163, 176
menopause/perimenopause 47–48
mermaids in wheelchairs 327
mess and confusion, starting with 173–175
metaphors 113, 113–114, 325–330
Michella, Monica 213
microbiome 55
micro-resting 153–154
micro-vision 274
Mindanao (Philippines), Tboli women 281
minimalism 222, 273
   continuum of maximalism and 21
mirrors 272
mistakes and errors 175–177
mixed media 311
mnemonics (memory aids) 183
mobility scooter 232, 244
modelling 311
Monet, Claude 24–25
mosaics 327
Mother Bear Project 317
motherhood 73–74, 104
motivation (and its deficiency) 23, 72, 221, 225
   reigniting 211
Moving Mountains 321–322
Mozart 49, 110
MRI Alchemist (Elizabeth Jameson) 26, 82
mud maid 327
multiple sclerosis (MS) 26, 82, 100, 285
muscles 163
   stretches 139–140
   use 137–138

Museum of International Folk Art 322
music 49–50, 58–59, 205–207, 311–312
   anxiety/depression and 58–59
   historical perspectives 28–29, 37–38
   piano 58–59, 75, 175, 183, 205–206, 214, 217–218
   rhythms 49, 240
myalgic encephalomyelitis (ME/CFS)
   author's onset in childhood 2
   help/information/resources 315, 319, 324
   people with 28, 29, 95, 97, 99, 124, 157, 163, 176, 178, 189, 217, 225, 278

nalbinding 191
narratives *see* stories/narratives
nature (and great outdoors) 85, 208, 268, 272, 312, 329–330
   Ovid on 154
   sounds 275
needle(s)
   knitting and crochet 66, 186–193
   sewing 193–198
   threaders/grabbers/pullers 193
needle felting 59, 198
needlework 313–314
negative space (*ma* - Japanese) 251, 253
nervous system
   neuroplasticity and 45–46
   parasympathetic 140
   sympathetic 53, 54, 141, 149
nests and 329
neuroplasticity 45–46, 49
neurotransmitters (brain) 55, 57, 129
Nightingale, Florence 277
Nightstand Collective 322
noise 136
novel-writing (fiction/stories) 28, 152–153, 165–166, 212
   flash fiction 109, 165, 281, 281

NumberSquares 81–82
Nye, Naomi Shihab (poet) 214

occupational therapy 41, 119, 162
O'Connor, Flannery 27–28
Octopus for a Preemie 317
Odin 329
O'Farrell, Lauren 83
online (internet) 286
    connections 92–93
    craftivism 83–84
    groups 93, 102, 178, 182
    list of resources 321–324
Online Art & Craft Club 322
origami butterflies 116–117
osmosis, absorbing by 285–286
others (other persons)
    borrowing from 285–289
    connecting with *see* connecting and connections
    helping 79–89
    learning from their path 34
Otter 302
outdoors *see* nature (and great outdoors)
Outside In 324
over-exertion 120, 143, 151, 155
overwhelming feelings 5, 60, 64
Ovid on nature 154

pacing 143–149
    finding your own pace 148–151
    pacing your learning 146–147
    from pushing to 143–159
    when pacing feels too hard 154–156
Paganini, Niccolo 29–30
pain
    aids/tools in management of 184
    conversation with 258
    when pushing 144
painting

negative space 253
past famous painters 24–26
tools/equipment/aids 198–201
see also artists; laughter painting; self-portrait
papercraft 162, 312
    cutting and tearing paper 59
    paper 59
parenthood 73–74, 104
past, reminiscing the 258
patchwork 63, 64, 74, 82, 195
    size considerations 164
path
    from author's to yours 1–6
    crafting your path 107–228
    learning from another's path 34
patient preparation 217–220
patterns, repetitive 240, 245
pencils 31, 51, 199, 200
pens 199, 201, 267
perceptions
    changing 231–236
    and widening of contradictory views 297
perennial plants 329
perfectionism 171–180
Perillo, Lucy 285
perimenopause 47–48
Perry, Grayson 222
Persephone 329
Persia, 11th century 39
personal agency 63, 64, 79, 300
personal significance 76
personal tension 127–133
Petals of Gratitude (UK) 317
Philippines, Tboli women 281
phoenix 327
photography/film/cameras 2, 204–205, 312
physical conditions *see* illness
physical space *see* space

Index

physiotherapy and mindful-based dance movement therapy 50
piano music 58–59, 75, 175, 183, 205–206, 214, 217–218
pilates 139–140
Pillow Crafters 322
Pillow Writers 322, 324
pinning 193–194
Pinterest 74, 322
pivot knitting 189
Pizza, Andy J 80–81
Plato 291
play and leisure time 120, 121, 157
    playing as practice 167–168
    see also entertainment
Plotnar, Jordan 82
poetry and poems 48, 165, 176–177, 203, 288
    fridge/magnetised boards 203
polymer clay 204
Portuguese knitting 188–189
Post Pals 315
postcards from another reality 282–283
postural tachycardia syndrome (PoTS) 50, 99
posture 137–138
pottery 204
power
    of community 94–98
    of you 88–89
practice (for creativity) 161–170
    commitment certificate 170
    good 161–170
    playing as 167–168
    preparation for see preparation
    shortcuts vs dead-ends 166–167, 258
praise 19
    unforthcoming 19–20
preparation for practice 161–163
    patient 217–220
prescriptions and prescribing 45–52
    social 42
present (current) moment 55–56, 258
pressure (psychological), dropping 129–130
pressure points (drawing) 133
Princess and the Pea 326
Procreate 200
productivity 70, 86, 143, 152
Project Linus UK 319
Proust, Marcel 266
pupae 329
purpose (meaning), sense of 69–77
pushing (incl. exertion) 143–159
    to pacing from 143–159
    when and when not to push 144–146
Pythagoras 38

quilting 164
    Love Quilts 318
    patchwork quilt 63, 74, 82, 164
    sensory quilt 218
quilting gloves 194

Rachel (ill person) 192
Rachel F. (ill person) 200
raised beds 208
Random Acts of Crochet Kindness UK 317
random connections 295–296
Rapunzel 326
Ravelry 74, 322
reaching 185–186
reclining 185–186
    Buddha statues 327
recorder (musical instrument) 206
relaxation 128, 140–141
religion, art and healing and 39–40
reminiscing the past 258
Ren (musician) 34
repetitive patterns and designs 240, 245

repetitive strain 191–192, 194
resilience, creating 64–65
Resonance Project 82, 319
rest *see* stopping
resting Buddha statues 327
Resting Up Collective 322
restrictions and limitations 21, 109
   of choice 123
   rhythms of 239–247
   wall (wall of illness) 4, 246
reward jar 158–159
rheumatoid arthritis 62
rhythms (rhythmic movements) 55, 239–247
   hands 37, 57
   music 49, 240
   restriction 239–247
Rilke, Rainer Maria 23, 257
Rip van Winkle 326
role (for yourself), creating 113–114
room (physical) *see* space
rotary cutter 194
Rumpelstiltskin 326
Ruth (ill person) 86

Sacks, Oliver 50
Sam (ill person) 63
Sanddancer Scarves for the Homeless 317
Sara (ill person) 31–32
satisfaction, choosing 278–279
scaling down 165
scent, following (exercise) 260–261
scissors 184, 194
Scottish knitters 189
screens (devices) 136, 201, 202
sculpting 46–47, 204
seasons, turning 241–242
seats *see* sitting
Sebold, Alice 269
Second World War 41, 267

The (Secret) Toy Society 319
seeds 329–330
self, inner 257–263
self-awareness 130, 236
self-censorship 251
self-criticism (inner critic) 171, 174, 178
self-denial 251, 254
self-esteem, low 64, 97
self-portrait 261
self-threading sewing needles 193
Selina (ill person) 58, 163, 176, 305
Selkies 326
sensations, paying attention to 136–137
sensory quilts 318
serotonin 57, 58
Sew Knit Crochet for the NHS and Charities 317, 319
sewing (incl. machine sewing) 193–198, 318–319
   size consideration 164
Sewing for Charity 318
shaky hands (tremors) 183, 200, 201
Shannan (ill person) 124
Shantel (ill person) 71
Shapiro, Francine 61
sharing stories 98–101, 299
Sharon (ill person) 199
sharpness of knitting needle 188
Shetland knitting belt 189
shortcuts 166–167
   inner path 258
shoulders 183–185
   dropping 128, 139
Sick 322–323
Siddal, Elizabeth 63
sighing, cyclic 140–141
significance, personal 76
silicone thimbles 188
simplifying your life 119–120
singing 93–94, 94, 206–207

Index

see also incantations
sitting (chairs and seats) 186
   gardening 207–208
   wheelchairs 185, 204, 208
size (of product) 164–166
S-J (ill person) 97, 337
Skillshare 322
sleep 280
   disorder (insomnia) 28, 181
Sleeping Beauty 326
Sleeping Hero (The King in the Mountain) 326
smartwatch 135
smell (sense of) (exercise) 260–261
Smith, Paul 26
snakes 330
social prescribing 42
solitude (aloneness and loneliness) 91–92, 95, 98, 101
songs *see* singing
Soul Treasures 225
sounds (paying attention to/listening to) 136
   of nature 275
space (physical), dedicated 123–124, 275
   sewing/beading/felting 194–195
   see also environment; negative space; white space
A Space Between 319
speech-to-text 201–202
spinning your own yarn 192–193
spirals 328–339
spontaneity 155, 161
Spoonie Press 323
square needle 186
star chart app 154
Stevenson, Robert Louis 34
Still Ill Ok 323
stillness 91, 157, 213, 218
stitch markers 190

Stitches of Support 317
Stitchlinks 323
stools 186
stopping (incl. rest/breaks/time-out) 144, 145, 147, 152–153, 156–158, 211, 215, 218, 224
   alternatives to 153–154
   enforced 221, 224
   struggling to know when to stop 151
stories/narratives (incl. lived experiences and other writings) 63, 299–306, 325–326
   guided visualisation aiding retrieval 303–305
   hidden/unexpressed stories 303
   sharing 98–101, 299
   see also novel-writing
stress
   brain and 140
   health and 53–55
stress hormones 66, 86, 131
Stuart-Smith, Sue 58
style, borrowing 287–288
suffering 72
suicide prevention 88
Sullivan, Glbert (cartoonist) 168
support *see* help and support
Surviving Severe ME 323
sustainability, maintaining a healthy sense of 130
sympathetic nervous system 53, 54, 141, 149

tapestry 196–197
tarot cards 328
Taylor-Bearman, Jessica 29
Tboli women of Mindanao (Philippines) 281
technology 92–93, 181–182
   drawing/painting 199–200
   written word 201–202

tension (personal) 127–133
textiles (incl. fabrics) 45–46, 313–314
    cutting 194–195
    drawing/painting 199–200
therapy
    mindful-based dance movement therapy 50
    occupational 41, 119, 162
    official emergence of art and craft therapy 41
thimbles 188
third hand tool 183
thirst, paying attention to 136–137
This is Colossal 323
thumb piano 205–206
Tibetan Buddhism 56
time management 151–153
tools/equipment/aids 22, 181–209
Toulouse-Lautrec, Henri de 242, 243
transformation 11, 12
trauma, alleviating 60–62
Trauma Teddies and Bobby Buddies 317
trees, deciduous 329
tremors (shaky hands) 183, 200, 201
trench art 267
tripod 205
triumphing over tragedy 71–72
tuberculosis 41
Tunisian crochet 191
Turner (artist) 215
turning seasons/year 241–242
twiddle muffs 318
Typewriter Artist (Paul Smith) 26

Ugly Duckling 326
Ukraine
    Kyiv 87
    Uzhhorod Hospital Donations Help Knit Crochet Craft Group 318
United By Wool – Helping Those in Need 318
upcycling 43, 257
usefulness of creativity 84–85

vagus nerve 50
van Gogh, Vincent 26
Versace, Donatella 291
Vi (ill person) 100
Viking crochet 191
visual art 40
    historical artists 24–27
visual imagery 327–328
visualisations 13, 257–258
    guided 303–305
Vivaldi, Antonio 29
voice of illness, listening to 265–270
voice-to-text 201–202
volunteering 101

Wade, Claire 28–29, 279
Walking 61, 244
wall of illness (restriction wall) 4, 246
Warm Baby Project 318
warning signs/alarm signs, body's 135, 143
Warrior Card Swap 315
watercolours 199
weather and internal weather 245–246
weaving 64
Weaving Loom 323
Western healthcare 40
wet-felting 197–198
wheelchairs 185, 204, 208, 244
white space 251
Whitney (ill person) 217
wind instrument 206
windows 271
Wishbone Words 323
Wood, Anna (ill person) 85
Woolf, Virginia 23, 174, 178
Woollen Woods 83–84

Index

Woolly Hugs 318
words 201–203, 314
    individuals' own words in a group 30–34
    see also writing
work, purpose 75
World War I and II 41, 267
The World Needs More Love Letters 315
'Would if I could' collage 254
Wounded/Fisher King 326
Write for Rights 315
Writers HQ 322–323
writing(s) 48–49, 201–203, 314, 325–326
    cathartic 37, 48
    expressive 48
    novels 28, 152–153, 165–166
    past famous writers 27–28
    see also words

yang and yin 296
yarns 47, 186, 188, 190–192, 221, 313–314
    guides and splitters 191
    tension 131
    see also crochet; knitting; sewing; weaving
Yarny Army 318
yin and yang 296
yoga 139–140
you, power of 88–89
YouTube 31, 218–229, 279
    tutorials 74, 181

Zausner, Tobi 24, 131, 242
zero-gravity space pens 201

Also from Hammersmith Health Books...

The Perrin Technique for ME/CFS and long COVID

Award-winning osteopath and leading authority on neuro-lymphatics, Raymond Perrin PhD has been researching the relationship between lymphatic drainage of the brain and energy levels – and putting this into clinical practice using The Perrin Technique – for over 30 years. Alerted to this essential connection when a patient recovered not only from back problems but also from ME/CFS symptoms, he shares the why and the how of the Perrin Technique in three outstanding guides:

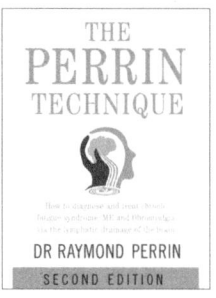

The Perrin Technique Second Edition: This illustrated guide for practitioners includes the underlying science that provides the rationale for the Perrin Technique's efficacy.
www.hammersmithbooks.co.uk/product/the-perrin-technique-2nd-edition/

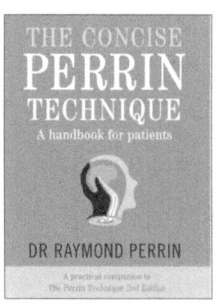

The Concise Perrin Technique: This is the guide for patients and their families who want the practical basics and a summary of the underlying science.
www.hammersmithbooks.co.uk/product/the-concise-perrin-technique/

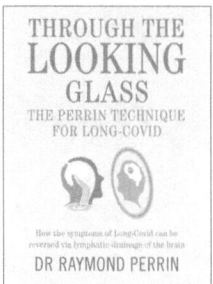

Through the Looking Glass: Dr Perrin's understanding of the neuro-lymphatic system led him to predict the epidemic of long COVID at the start to the COVID-19 pandemic. Here he explains the underlying disease mechanisms of that condition and how the Perrin Technique can reverse the condition.
www.hammersmithbooks.co.uk/product/through-the-looking-glass/

Also from Hammersmith Health Books…

Diagnosis and Treatment of Chronic Fatigue Syndrome, Myalgic Encephalitis and Long COVID
It's mitochondria, not hypochondria
Third edition

By Dr Sarah Myhill and Craig Robinson

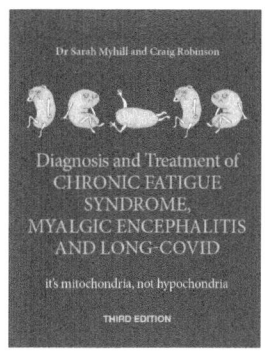

Since the publication of its first edition in April 2014, Dr Myhill's guide to understanding and overcoming CFS/ME has become a must-read for sufferers from this poorly understood condition. With its focus on promoting the health of our mitochondria – the power-houses of our cells – with the right diet, supplements and lifestyle measures while addressing the factors that destroy our mitochondria – including toxins, chronic infections, stress and other emotional problems – we can find a clear path to improving our energy levels. Dr Myhill, supported by expert patient Craig Robinson, emphasises what we can do for ourselves as efficiently and cost-effectively as possible.

www.hammersmithbooks.co.uk/product/diagnosis-and-treatment-of-chronic-fatigue-syndrome-myalgic-encephalitis-and-long-covid-third-edition/

Also from Hammersmith Health Books...

Fighting Fatigue
A practical guide to managing the symptoms of CFS/ME

Edited by Sue Pemberton and Catherine Berry

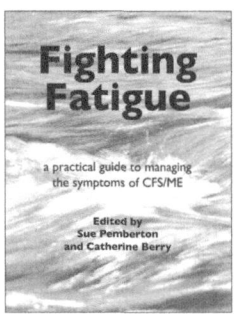

Written by a collaboration of occupational therapists and recovered CFS/ME patients, this is now the standard text for pacing during recovery. With energy levels fluctuating wildly – the 'boom and bust' pattern typical of CFS/ME – you may well feel stuck in a downward spiral of setbacks and relapse. Yet it is this cycle of boom and bust that Fighting Fatigue aims to help you not only break but also use to support your recovery.

www.hammersmithbooks.co.uk/product/fighting-fatigue/

Also from Hammersmith Health Books…

The Fatigue Book
Chronic fatigue syndrome and long COVID fatigue: practical tips for recovery

By Lydia Rolley

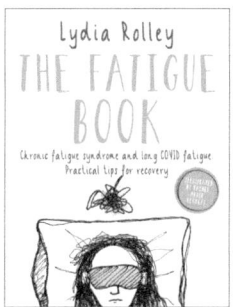

This is a practical, attractively illustrated guide to managing CFS/ME and long COVID in order to enable recovery at a pace that works for the individual. Whether someone is at the start of their recovery journey or has been doing this for some time, there is clear, practical advice based on a self-management approach that applies the principles of Pacing and Activity Management (but NOT Graded Exercise), as recommended by the new NICE guidelines for both conditions. Each chapter includes a range of Tips from which to choose plus Food for thought, Pause and Mind, body and soul. Essential text is highlighted so that the severely fatigued can focus purely on that in the early stages of recovery.

www.hammersmithbooks.co.uk/product/the-fatigue-book/

Also from Hammersmith Health Books…

Rest-Do Days
Now to live with fatigue and get things done

By Wendy Bryant

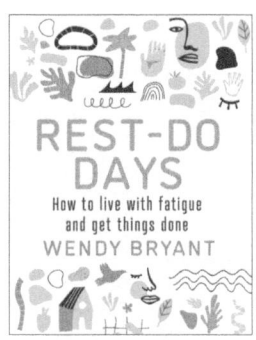

A practical guide to finding a balance between resting and doing so that readers can recharge their energy levels and also do the things that are important to them. Using concepts from occupational therapy about pacing, occupational balance and creativity in everyday life, this approach is based on the Author's professional experience as an occupational therapist and her personal experience of living with chronic illness through which she has learned how to adapt her rest-activity balance, keeping an eye on what (or who) is controlling her decisions and focusing on doing what's important and satisfying in her life.

www.hammersmithbooks.co.uk/product/rest-do-days-how-to-live-with-fatigue-and-get-things-done/